DESTRESS TO SUCCESS

Solving Stress and Winning Big in
Relationships, Wealth and Life Itself

By Leo Willcocks

DESTRESS TO SUCCESS

Solving Stress and Winning Big in
Relationships, Wealth and Life Itself

Disclaimer

The information provided in this book is designed to provide helpful information on the subjects discussed. This book is not meant to be used, nor is it be used, to diagnose or treat any medical or psychiatric condition. For diagnosis or treatment of any medical or psychiatric problem, consult your own physician.

The publisher and author are not responsible for any specific medical or health needs that may require supervision by a licensed healthcare practitioner, and thus they are not liable for any consequences from any recommendation to any person reading or following the information in this book.

Neither the publisher nor the author shall be liable for any loss of profit or any other commercial damages, including but not limited to special, incidental, consequential, or other damages.

Innovation Publishing
Las Vegas, Nevada, USA
(702) 997 2229

In Praise of DeStress To Success by Leo Willcocks:

"*DeStress to Success* is the gift that keeps on giving, from specific situations to long-term solutions. If you have ever felt stressed–and who hasn't–Leo Willcocks offers a terrific new perspective on keeping calm."

–Harvey Mackay
Author of the #1 New York Times bestseller
Swim With The Sharks Without Being Eaten Alive

"This book shows you how to achieve inner peace, happiness and a calm effective attitude toward life."

–Brian Tracy
CEO, Top selling author of over 45 books and
over 300 programs including the best-selling
Psychology of Achievement

"*DeStress to Success* offers real, working solutions for coping with stress. Filled with effective strategies and tools, this book shows you how to find the peace and perspective you crave in order to live a life of greater contribution and less stress."

-Stephen M. R. Covey
Author of The New York Times and
1 Wall Street Journal bestseller,
The Speed of Trust, and co-author of *Smart Trust*

"Human beings are hardwired to achieve greatness. Lack of confidence in our abilities, for whatever reason, creates the stress that holds us back. In *DeStress to Success*, Leo Willcocks shows us simple, yet powerful, strategies for unleashing our greatest potential. Read it today!"

-Tom Hopkins
Bestselling author of *How to Master the Art of Selling*

"If you want a real solution for stress, then *DeStress to Success* is the book for you. Leo Willcocks lays it all out on the table, with practical solutions to relieve and solve stress."

-Robert G. Allen
International Multi-bestselling author
Creating Wealth, Multiple Streams of Income, Multiple Streams of Internet Income, Nothing Down, Nothing Down for Women, The One Minute Millionaire, Cracking the Millionaire Code, and *Cash in a Flash.*

"*DeStress to Success* is a wonderful, values-based book that not only helps you solve stress in your life, but will also show you how to live a more enjoyable and happier life, experience improved relationships with those you love, and help you find success in your work and all aspects of life. It is a must read for all who want more happiness, less stress and greater meaning in their lives."

-W. Steve Albrecht
Awarded in the Top 50 Corporate Directors,
National Association of Corporate Directors;
author, professor, church leader

"If you want less stress and more happiness in your life, then *DeStress to Success* delivers!"

- Sean Covey
Bestselling author of *The 7 Habits of Highly Effective Teens*

"The practical information in *DeStress to Success* will open your eyes to a life with less stress and more satisfaction and peace."

-Doug Wead
Bestselling author, speaker and former advisor
to the Bush White house

"*DeStress to Success* empowers you to rise above the sources of stress in your life and turn the very challenges that cause stress into the seeds of greater success, happiness and fulfillment."

-Dr. Denis Waitley
Bestselling author of *The Seeds of Greatness*

"In the high-tech, 24/7 world in which we live, learning to deal with stress is the key to business and personal success. Through examples and stories, Willcocks shows us what causes stress, and he provides easy-to implement strategies to help anyone find inner peace."

-**Sam Richter**
Bestselling and award-winning author
and top-ranked international speaker

"If you feel that stress is controlling your life, then *DeStress to Success* is for you. It puts you back in the driver's seat of life, letting you - and not the stressful situations and circumstances around you - make the calls."

-**Stefanie Hartman**
Marketing strategist, TV host, creator of the
Stop Trading Your Time for Money™

"Anyone who has ever known the debilitation of anxiety and worry should own this book. Leo Willcocks delivers the tools so you never have to feel that way again. You can take control and strip back to the core issues that have been playing havoc with your emotions, fix them, and enjoy a life filled with success and joy from within!"

-**Cydney O'Sullivan**
International Best Selling Author of *How to Be Wealthy NOW!* And
Social Marketing Superstars: Social Media Mystery to Mastery in 30 Days

Bonuses

Bonus Resources

I can't give you everything you need to know about stress in one book (even though I have packed as many stress resolving tools into *DeStress to Success* as possible), so I have created a website with special gifts to help quickly reduce your stress. In it you'll find:

> ➤ The *Am I Stressed*? checklist to help you find your true stress levels
> ➤ My Stress Mapping tool to help you identify:
>> ➤ the main areas of stress in your life
>> ➤ where that stress is coming from
>> ➤ your path to less stress
> ➤ Step-by-step training modules to walk you through key stress reduction tools in *DeStress to Success*
> ➤ Insightful articles and resources to help you have more peace and enjoyment in life

To access these valuable gifts, visit
http://www.leowillcocks.com/bookgifts.html

For all of those seeking relief from stress—
from the overworked executive to
the work-from-home parent,
and everyone they meet along the way.

TABLE OF CONTENTS

Introduction 1

Chapter 1: Where Does Stress Come From? 5

Chapter 2: Seeing Both Sides 23

Chapter 3: Stress and the Natural Relationship Cycle 52

Chapter 4: How Relationships Generate Stress 69

Chapter 5: Deep, Lasting Love: The Fortified Relationship 99

Chapter 6: The Workplace 123

Chapter 7: Your Money or Your Life: Stress and Finances 156

Chapter 8: Moving Into Self-Love 182

Chapter 9: Conquering Fear & Stress 202

Chapter 10: Peace from Within 221

Final Word 236

References and bibliography 237

Introduction

We all want a life without stress. A life where we feel fulfilled and on purpose each day, where we enjoy sunny days, blue skies and rainbows. A life where our confidence and peace of mind emanate like sunrise over the beach. Where minor ups and downs have no effect on our stress levels whatsoever. A life where, if challenges do occur, we are calm, wise, and emerge victorious, and our lives are even better from the experience. We all want to enjoy the good in life without stress getting in our way.

While a life with *no* stress is really an illusion, we can have *far less* stress in our lives. In fact, often our greatest sources of stress can be resolved. So, how do we move beyond the daily bombardment of stress and into more peace?

The first step is to change our approach to stress. Stress is something that most of us accept as part of life. As a general rule, however, most of us accept it too much. We are so used to it that we usually don't even notice it happening. We carry on, living each day with varying levels of stress, without even realizing what we're experiencing. When something goes wrong - like someone cutting us off in traffic, being in the 'slow line' in the grocery store, or a child or our partner doing something we don't like - our primitive stress responses of anger and fear kick into gear. These reactions can be loud and rather inflammatory, and usually don't end well. Even at this point, when all this is happening, we don't think that we are stressed - we usually think it is all the other person's fault.

Aside from reacting with anger or fear, another common way we respond is to make like an ostrich: stick our head in the sand and hope it passes by. We might talk about our situation with family or friends. We probably try and relieve or ignore it with alcohol, food, chocolate, and entertainment. But in terms of acting to solve the problem, our head goes in the sand. Instead, we mask the feeling of stress because inwardly, either we don't feel capable of resolving the challenge, or we think that it is a normal part of life and there isn't any other way.

This cycle of reacting and ignoring doesn't solve our problems or stress - it helps them get worse. Just like a car gradually falls into disrepair if we don't get an oil change and fix minor problems as they occur, our "stresses" can gradually fester, especially when our anger reactions contribute. If this carries on long enough, disaster can follow. Relationships end. Work productivity goes down and performance reviews look bad. Children rebel. Financial challenges reach a breaking point. And one day or another, we step back and think "What happened? What went wrong?"

But there is another way - a better way. We *can* rise above stress. We don't have to be at the mercy of life's circumstances when it comes to stress. We can have the confidence, calmness and peace of mind we want. We can have complete mental relief (both immediate and long term) from the frustrations and cares we feel. We can have the clarity and wisdom to deal with challenges in ways that create happiness. We can become resilient to stress, so we are less likely to become overwhelmed by life's big and small challenges. Day by day, bit by bit, we can become stress proof.

The Problem with Modern Day Stress Relief

The problem with modern day stress relief is that its main arsenal is stress relief tips. These tips are great at giving short term relief of stress. You feel better, you are more focused. The problem that was causing you panic seems more manageable, and not so bad after all. You are more able to carry on enjoying your day, and you can act to resolve challenges from a more calm state of mind.

This is all we need, right? Wrong. While this is all great, the problem is that it is all temporary, eventually the stress returns, like a mother bear returning to her cubs when a threat is near. This can happen days, weeks, hours, or even minutes after our walk, massage, yoga routine, exercise, or meditation. It's like you never did anything to relieve stress in the first place. What do you do then?

Another problem is that it isn't always practical. You can't exactly bust out in yoga poses when your manager is giving out orders. You can't necessarily go for a walk when your toddler or teenager is having a tantrum in a public place. And you may not have the hours needed to develop Zen monk focus. So what do you do then?

In some ways, most of the stress relief techniques out there are just much better versions of masking and ignoring stress. They are better because they don't have bad health effects (like alcohol), they do temporarily give us more clarity of mind, and they also have long term benefits in terms of health and well-being. But you tell me, is this enough?

We need something powerful. Something just as good at immediately relieving stress as modern stress relief tips - but better. We need something that lasts longer, so we stay calm, and the stress doesn't return. We also need something that can be done discreetly, without anyone knowing.

The Stress Puzzle

Stress relief tips are just one piece of the stress puzzle. If we want:

- short and long term stress relief,
- to be calm and not react in stressful situations,
- to be unperturbed by challenges and not become stressed in the first place,
- more happiness and peace of mind,

- more satisfaction and success - in our relationships, personal and professional endeavors,

To be really free of stress's frustrating influence in our lives, we need all of the pieces to this puzzle. Without these pieces, we stay stuck in the react-ignore cycle, experiencing the downs of life far more than we want.

There is already a wealth of information available on stress relief tips. Because of this, I have chosen to focus on the pieces of the puzzle you don't already have. In this book, I have included very powerful techniques that will give you that instant relief you are looking for, as well as those missing pieces of the puzzle that will make the biggest difference. You will learn:

- Heat of the moment, stress-dissolving techniques that have immediate benefits, but also reduce your long term stress levels
- How to disengage your anger and fear response when stresses occur
- A deeper understanding of the causes of stress in your own life
- How to prevent several common and major stresses from occurring
- How to lower your susceptibility to stress and increase your resilience
- How to do all this without sacrificing hours of your time

The fact that you are here, reading this book, is an indicator that you are already on your way. You want more than to have stress as a common thread throughout your life. You are willing to go beyond the react-ignore cycle, and you are ready to put in the relatively small amount of effort needed. You are ready to DeStress.

Chapter 1: Where Does Stress Come From?

Imagine taking an excursion into the Amazon River basin. You and your friends board a boat in Iquitos, the main Peruvian river port, and cruise for a few hours, intently aware of the scenery around you. Then you detour into the Yanayacu River, a tributary, and from there into smaller tributaries. All have their own features and microclimates, their rainforest canopies, exotic delights and their dangers; all demand your rapt attention. When you cruise back, your boat increases speed as one tributary pours into the other, en route to the mile-wide Amazon, which moves swiftly toward the Atlantic. Now imagine being lifted out of this tiny section of the Amazon. As you ascend, you see more and more tributaries, spreading in all directions, until it looks like the arteries, veins and capillaries of your cardiovascular system. You may see thousands of sources that feed the Amazon. The mighty river takes it all in, building pressure and intensity, sweeping up more and more flotsam, widening and sometimes flooding its banks. Finally, it spills into the Atlantic through a delta that is 200 miles wide.

If you were to make a 3D model of the collective causes of stress in the 19th or early 20th century, the model would be no larger than a couple of tributaries and the main river. There were stressors, but in simpler times came more acceptance of situations as they existed. People didn't stress out over the little things. Today, however, the sources of your stress or mine might look like the entire Amazon River watershed. Causes feed other causes, which multiply into more triggers, flooding our dreams and willpower, and finally sweeping pieces of our lives into a place of endless depth from where it's very hard to retrieve them.

Try a simple experiment. Next time you are in a sizable city, say 200,000 or more people, stand on an intersection for fifteen minutes. Tune in with your senses, and absorb every sensation that comes your way. *Everything.* How do you feel? Nervous?

Overwhelmed? Electrified? Now imagine that each sensation produces some sort of stress in your body or mind (maybe you don't have to imagine that at all!). Stressors come from everywhere –different cars, buildings, billboards, shouts of bystanders, food stands. Finally, like tributaries, they come together to create an overwhelming situation – your body and mind in a stressed-out state.

What Causes Stress?

What causes stress in your life? What are the contributing factors? Events? Interactions that make you nervous or uptight? Which people? What activities? What times of year? And how do they affect your greatest right in this life–the right to love yourself? In order to study the ways in which stress affects us, and how we can minimize, reduce and eliminate stress from our lives, we need to know where the stress comes from. We need to backtrack to the origination points. We need to rewind all the way back to see how our day began, what set us up to be stressed, and what caused us to react to some sensations harshly and others not at all.

In my work, I have learned that many of our stresses, struggles and emotional challenges are also rooted somewhere in our childhoods. Every time a stressful or challenging situation reminds us, consciously or subconsciously, of a damaging incident in childhood, the toxic imprint of that event pulses outward like a solar flare. It burns into our perception, causing us to behave in the same way, react as we did at age ten, or fall into a bad habit. We have to go back to the beginning to pinpoint the stressors in our lives, and work through them so we don't respond with knee-jerk, defensive reactions that add to the problem. Looking at our childhoods is one way of reviewing where our stress comes from. In all, there are five areas we will explore in this chapter:

1. Outside sources: environmental, modern society, lifestyle
2. Cause and effect
3. Fear
4. Childhood demons
5. Nutritional deficiencies or hormone imbalances

Once we figure out the causes of our stress, we can take action to minimize or remove them from our lives. The trick is to figure them out. Let's take a look at these causes. Note in your mind (or a piece of paper) which of these might apply to you.

Outside Sources

Modern society makes it difficult to give enough "quality time" to our family, work, personal growth, and recreational time. Consequently, some things fall by the wayside. Our health may deteriorate as we spend less and less time exercising and eating right. Our family might suffer if we don't give time to them. We may miss out on a good promotion from not putting in extra effort at work. But we have to keep up with that schedule, the kids' homework, the yard, our finances … our relationships. There are just too many things to do!

Out of this hamster wheel of responsibility and expectation comes a variety of situations. Each can ratchet up stress, but most people carry around a combination of:

o "Keeping up with the Joneses"
o Ambition
o Hell bent determination to achieve perceived norms or goals at all costs
o Career change

o Workplace problems
o Job dissatisfaction
o Relationship problems
o Family problems
o Dietary problems
o Addictions, in varied forms: drugs, alcohol, sex, gambling, etc.
o Health concerns

What's a Stressor? What Is Stress? What's the Difference?

When we feel stressed, the natural reaction is to blame the stressful event for our frustration, anger or upset. How many times have you heard the words, "You make me feel ____" "Stop making me _____"?

In reality, the stressor–the event, action or circumstance–and the internal stress response you feel are two different things. When you mentally separate the two, you are more in control of your stress, instead of it being in control of you. The reason we so easily blame one event for all of our feelings of stress is partially because of our societal tendency to take an attitude of "She'll be right, mate." That is, we keep pushing forward as if the problems and stressors aren't there. We carry on as much as we can without dealing with a stressful situation. It may seem too hard to address, or just be easier to not do anything about it. We might complain about it to friends and family, but not act to correct the situation. Eventually, it takes its toll. Our stress levels get to the point that we become run down. We snap at family or co-workers. We yell at those who cut us off in traffic, and may even use hand gestures to emphasize our point. The simple ups and downs of life frustrate us.

One way of looking at this is to imagine your stress levels like a pot of boiling water. When the water in your pot and your residual stress levels are low, you are more capable of dealing with ups and downs. You can see situations more clearly. You don't get aggravated so easily. However, as the days, weeks or months go on, and stresses pour in from the sources discussed in this chapter, the water levels in your pot start to rise. Big challenges add large amounts of water. Sometimes, your level drops when a challenge is resolved. Sometimes, the water levels remain high.

When the boiling water is almost at the top, you feel the effect of stress. You are easily aggravated. The demands of your time and energy bog you down. You are snappy, and see the bad side of things. Your shoulders, neck or jaw may be tense and painful. You may notice that your 'frown lines' seem deeper than before. You may become more reliant on alcohol or cigarettes to 'relax'. In this state, all it takes is one little event to make your pot boil over. You react. Hot water and steam burst out, burning anyone close enough. When these events happen, it really feels like that one current problem has caused all of your stress. Commonly, we blame that particular, in-the-moment situation, just like the little mouse is blamed for sinking the boat in Pamela Allen's famous "Who Sank the Boat?" We direct our stress reaction at that problem, person, or event. It's their fault after all – or so it feels!

In reality, this is not the case. You are reacting with frustration, anger, and other feelings that have been stewing for some time. Your feelings of stress, and your reaction, result from a full pot of boiling water, not the last ounce or two that overflowed. The resulting feelings and reactions are often blown completely out of proportion with the current event. Have you ever looked back in hindsight and thought "I took that a little too far"? Or, "I blew that out of proportion"? At the time it didn't feel that way though, did it?

Another way to think of this is the phrase, "The straw that broke the camel's back." It comes from the idea that a camel carries more and more straw, until one last straw is placed. The combined weight breaks the camel's back, but only the last straw took the load from manageable to too much. One of the core practices we will discuss and explore in this book is how to recognize that last straw *before* you put it on your back–and from there, how to never carry such a full load that your sanity and well-being comes down to one straw.

Many of us are used to constantly living with our water levels boiling close to the top. We don't even notice that constant feeling of stress anymore; we are used to it. We may even think it is normal. There is, however, a solution. There is another way! This book is full of answers for reducing those residual water levels. But first we must learn what to do in those boiling over situations.

One helpful step is to realize that our feelings of stress and the event itself are two separate things. We can control our stress response, no matter how bad the situation seems. That last event, no matter how big, is most likely not responsible for all of those current feelings of stress. The following questions will help increase your awareness of the contributors to your "pot". When you mentally acknowledge that other factors besides the current event contribute to your feeling of stress, you are more able to respond calmly and constructively. Ask yourself:

1. Why am I really stressed?
2. How did I feel before this happened? What other events could be contributing to how I feel right now?
3. Are my reactions and feelings on par with what is happening right now? Or are they also because of previous events?
4. Recognize that the current situation is not as bad as it seems or feels.
5. Ask yourself: What would be a good way that I can handle this situation?
6. Work on the current situation. Give yourself permission to postpone your stress about other frustrations.

7. At a better time, consider appropriate ways to handle the other situations contributing to your stress.

The goal of these questions is not for you to dwell on all of your stresses at once. If you start to dwell, stop. Instead, recognize that your stress comes from a variety of events or situations, and take proactive action at the appropriate time to resolve each challenge. Focus on the one current event now.

Cause and Effect

Stress occurs from cause and effect. It begins with our attitude toward any given situation or relationship. Our attitudes can cause stress. We stress ourselves by creating overly high expectations, and then trying to live up to those expectations of ourselves and others. Even if well intended, this attitude can really hurt us. Furthermore, I see an increasingly more prevalent attitude among clients and others that "the world owes me". For some reason, we expect others to be responsible for our happiness – our parents, bosses, friends, colleagues or governments. This is not the road to a stress-free life.

Every time we take an action that involves another person, or a group of people, it affects that person or group in some way. Likewise, when they take an action that involves you, it will affect you–positively or negatively. Question is, do those actions add to your stress? Or reduce it? A very interesting take on this subject comes from people who have written about near-death experiences and their specific experiences in that state. One, by *A Taste of Eternity* author Martha Halda, discussed something very distinctive that happened during a near-death experience following an almost fatal car crash in 1999–the impact of her actions, feelings and words toward others. "Not only did I have to feel the positives and negatives of my own actions, but I had to feel how they affected the other person–exactly how they felt at the time," she wrote. "So if I hurt them, suddenly, I was hurting.

Intensely. If I caused them stress, I suddenly felt totally stressed out. It is something I never want to feel again."

Every action you take on your own, without others' involvement, will impact your next moment positively or negatively. It will either add to or reduce the stress in your life. If you eat unhealthy food and never exercise, your fitness will drop. When you do that enough times, over enough years, you may have a heart attack, diabetes, early-onset dementia, or a stroke. This is especially true if your family history predisposes you to specific diseases or ailments. Such a health crisis, along with not being able to work and the financial pressure of hospital bills, becomes very stressful.

Another cause and effect relationship is over prioritizing work at the expense of your partner and/or children. In time, they may feel disconnected from you. Your children may rebel against your authority, or take wrongful actions that causes you stress. They may rebel because you've lost the ability to communicate with them or to better understand their worlds (not that we ever fully do!). For those and other reasons, you may have relationship problems with your partner that result in strained communication, broken promises (like vacations that have to be postponed or cancelled), reduced sexual relations, and other forms of internal strife that lead to broken marriages or relationships—and estranged relationships with children.

Another example comes from not setting personal boundaries. Your coworkers may take you for granted and ask you to do extra things for which they are responsible. Your boss might expect you to always rise above and beyond the call of duty (without any increase in pay). You could end up never receiving what you want in your friendships or relationships, because you are always trying to please others. You always let them have what they want—and they feel no obligation or desire to return the favor. In time, those friends without respect or common decency run over you, pouring right through your hopes or desires. Whose choice is that? Theirs to run over you?

Or yours to let it happen? You chose not to bury a foot in the sand and say, "Not this time. I won't let you go beyond this point." In a way, the ensuing stress you feel over never being heard or respected is an effect of your own behavior and decision to not set personal boundaries.

Just as specific actions cause stress, other specific actions resolve stress and create peace and pleasure in life. Throughout the coming chapters you will find a multitude of actions that help resolve specific stressors and create peace.

Fear

Fear is the double-edged sword of stress. Not only does a lot of our stress come from fearful situations, or the things we fear, but when we project that fear, it produces even more stress. Quick case in point: In 2013 in Los Angeles, a rogue cop, Christopher Dorner, went on his own personal manhunt against other cops. On the day the week-long drama came to an end, he broke into a cabin in the Southern California mountains, and tied up a couple – but didn't hurt them. He never hurt any civilians; only cops. When interviewed a month after the incident, one of the tied-up victims said she still couldn't sleep well. Her nightmares felt like real life, and she refused to walk into her cabin. That's the double-edged relationship between fear and stress. Obviously, being tied up by a cop killer on the run is a stressor of the highest level. It is also most every person's deepest fear. It's what happened *afterward,* the post-traumatic stress that is the debilitating product of the fear-stress relationship. She expected another intruder to tie her up. She never turned off the lights. Her lack of sleep caused over-anxiety and the strange thoughts that accompany insomnia. She wouldn't go home; she and her husband lived from place to place, from relative's house to relative's house. It makes people cringe when they hear about it. Her life was like watching an intense horror film, wondering what would pop out to terrify her next. This is an extreme example, however many of us experience this fear in smaller degrees during every day events.

I focus on fear in a later chapter, so I won't elaborate much at this point, other than to review how fear it feeds stress. Sometimes, we associate a specific situation with a negative outcome. For example, do you like being stuck in traffic? It can make you run late, you must listen to complaining children or teenagers while cooped up together in the car, other people blast their horns repeatedly, and you envision the people at work, or your spouse at home, pacing back and forth, peeking at their watches, wondering where on Earth you are. Furthermore, you *know* you're going to catch hell for it when you arrive. You fear being late and hearing about it, the type of fear that elevates the heartbeat and your irritability simultaneously. All you wanted was to get to your destination without a traffic jam to foul up the day!

Most likely, when a situation like this happens again, but you *aren't* running late, you will still feel stressed. Why? Because neurons that fire together wire together, and your brain has associated heavy traffic with all the negative outcomes from past traffic experiences, activating your stress response. The frustration and fear you felt in those stressful situations, automatically surfaces again - even when you are not late, and you won't have those negative outcomes. But the stress still happens, doesn't it? This is another reason why our stress response can be beyond the severity of the stressful event itself.

Another fear-based stressor that we have all experienced, more times than we like, concerns finances. What if we can't pay our bills? How will we pay the mortgage? What do we do now that you, or I, have lost our jobs? How do I save for the kids' college *and* take care of the home remodel we desperately need *and* help out my elderly parents? How do I afford any of this? How do I keep earning income when the information technology economy has sucked away my secretarial job at a smelting plant? If anything could be identified as the leading cause of mass social and personal stress since the global economy withdrew into deep recession in 2008, this would likely be it.

Stress pours directly from fear-based questions like those above. When reading this paragraph, for example, did you feel yourself seize up a little? Remember what I said just a minute ago: *neurons that fire together wire together.* Unless you are an emotional giant who can stop the momentum from snowballing, it will lead to another stress. And another. And then some fear. Followed by more stress. Soon, the stress is monumental, blown way out of proportion compared to the single event, or question that caused it in the first place. Only problem is, *you* don't see this. And you're the one feeling it.

Childhood Demons

People are often not aware of this source of stress, but it may be responsible for a lot of the problems with which they deal presently. Therefore, resolving this stress by exploring our childhood demons can be the most helpful. People have a much more difficult time pinpointing their causes of stress when it relates to their childhood. At the same time, dealing with these challenges can be the most empowering. You will incur stress-producing situations on a regular basis that come from a present, current event (what I call a "now" event), working too many hours, for example. Others may arise from the recurrence of deep rooted problems learned or carried on from the past - someone confronts you in a particularly angry tone, and instead of diffusing the situation, you push back hard, and create the same situation that caused you untold problems on the school playground.

Many situations will combine current challenges and childhood demons. Often, the current situation is a trigger that unearths a deep-rooted cause of stress, although you might have no perspective of that, as the event is actually unfolding. The current situation grows more stressful because of the deep-rooted problem.

Let me share an experience with a client. She was getting angry about the things people said when they were not minding their own business – a "now" event. In addition, they were being rude about the way she did things, even when her actions did not concern them. We stress when someone is gossiping maliciously about us. Now imagine that happening to someone as emotionally sensitive as my client – in the middle of one busy workday after another. This situation brought her face to face with a childhood demon, a persistent cause of stress. As a child, she learned to be quiet when people were aggressive, and never learned to be assertive or set boundaries (for fear of physical retribution). But now, years later, she still allowed other people to overpower her. This became so frustrating that she would get angry and take it out on her family – but never on the people actually overpowering her.

If she already knew how to be assertive, the current situation would not be that stressful. But the inherent fear of setting boundaries–because of her past trauma–caused her near-paralytic stress. This set up the next stage of a damaging cause-and-effect cycle: because she didn't set boundaries, others held no respect toward her. She constantly resented them, and felt powerless to change the situation. My client let people run over her for years before she couldn't take it anymore, and came to see me.

Another way of thinking of her situation – and, for that matter, unreleased stress – is like a volcano. Just as pressure builds from deep within the Earth's surface, our stress is often found deep below the surface of our lives. The "magma" and "gases" of stress might have pooled up 20, 30 or 50 years ago. In other words, our volcano has been dormant for years, maybe decades. Then it begins to billow. The "magma" is all the accumulated stress, tension and baggage. But it goes unnoticed. Then a specific situation triggers an eruption – the straw that broke the camel's back. All magma from the past rushes up and out, turning life into a virtual Pompeii, where you feel buried alive in the course of an hour. You blame the situation that tipped you over the edge. But the true problem lies beneath the volcano: the deeply rooted stress. For my client, the trigger situation was the aggressive coworker not minding her own business. The underlying problem, however, was her lack of knowing how to be assertive, compounded by the greater fear of standing up for herself. The magma contained the fear, frustration and pain experienced in her traumatic childhood, where she learned to be passive, as well as the frustration from her current trigger experience. She had to recognize each situation that required her assertiveness, learn how to be assertive without being angrily confrontational, and learn how to face and overcome traumatic situations in a far different way than she did in her past.

Without learning how to overcome deeply rooted stresses, it is common to cycle through the same problems again and again. For many people, this means having recurring relationship problems with each new partner. Or ending up with jobs that are not fulfilling–over and over again. When you are feeling stressed, it helps to recognize if there is a deeper reason behind your stress. You can become more aware and less affected by the current frustration. You can release frustration and approach the situation with a clearer frame of mind. Ask yourself these questions when feeling stressed:

- o "Why am I really stressed?"
- o Think of the answer and ask: "Why does that bother me?"
- o When you have the answer to the second question, again ask yourself: "Why does that (the second answer) bother me?"

Answering these questions will help you recognize other factors impacting your stress levels about the situation, and deeper reasons for your stress. Then to really drive it home and uncover the deep volcanoes–the ones which have the biggest influence on your frame of mind now–ask yourself:

- o "Has this situation, or a similar one, ever happened before?"
- o "How do I feel about that previous situation? "Do I have any anger or upset?"
- o "Could any of that stress be influencing how I feel now?"

Most often, past unresolved stress is carried on to future similar situations.

As you work with this, don't allow yourself to dwell on past events. Keep an eye on our goal in this book: being stressed is not going to help the situation at all. If anything, it will impact us in a negative way. We may not think of answers to the situations; at the very least, our solutions will be far less creative or possible. When we feel stressed, we experience more activity in the emotion area and primitive response areas of our brains. These are our survival centers–fight or flight. This means we react more. Simultaneously, we also have less activity in the thought and planning areas of the brain, meaning it is harder to see the answer to the problem. However, if you use these questions correctly, you will be able to rein in that stress response. You will feel more capable of handling the current situation, and learning from past experiences.

Nutritional Deficiencies or Hormonal Imbalances

In America, a refrigerator magnet made the rounds a few years ago, as the fight between organic growers and genetically modified seed producers, such as Monsanto, kicked into high gear. It read, "Eat Organic Food – Or As Your Grandparents Called It, 'Food'."

There is a lot to this saying. Agribusiness, fertilizer, herbicides, pesticides and their use by global farmers skyrocketed after World War II. Yes, food production worldwide soared, but so did meat consumption (85% of all corn and soybeans grown in the U.S. feeds cows, pigs and other sources of meat worldwide, according to the Department of Agriculture). Along with agribusiness came the effects of all the chemicals–disease, anxiety-related disorders, increased chronic ailments such as diabetes, hormonal imbalances (particularly among teenage girls and women balancing work and families), and diets became far less nutritious than those our grandparents ate. There is more food, but far less nutritious food. That's the price of agribusiness.

When you combine that reality with our fast-paced lives, in which few people eat three square meals a day, but the majority eat junk food at least twice per week, you arrive at what I believe to be a dangerous situation: nutritional deficiencies and hormonal imbalances among people racing around in their lives and burning more energy than they take in through food… The result? A constant feeling of being stressed, nervous, anxious and tense. Put these contributing factors together, and it is one reason why hypertension and stress-based disorders in industrialized nations have increased by *more than 500 percent* since 1950, according to the U.S. Center for Disease Control.

You can take very direct steps to alleviate the additional stress and unhealthiness caused by a poor diet or hormonal imbalance. *Change your diet.* Eat more fruits and vegetables, and some particular root vegetables (yams, beets, turnips, etc.) that are alkaline and diminish stress. Cut back on white foods (pasta, white bread, white rice, etc.) and opt for grains that combine protein and carbohydrates (quinoa, buckwheat, brown rice, etc.). Eat less meat and more fish, or meat substitutes such as beans. Also, if you can, make lunch your primary meal, with lighter but equally nutritious breakfasts and dinners. Or, break it up into five small meals per day. And take supplements–at least a multi-vitamin, and something to reduce stress, such as salmon oil capsules. By doing this, you will feel stronger and healthier, and your energy level will increase. The more energy you feel, the harder it is for stress to take hold. Plus, you will feel better, and have a more positive, proactive attitude when dealing with potentially stressful situations. When your nutrition increases, it tends to help with hormonal imbalance as well.

Minimizing and Alleviating Stress–And Turning It Around

In reality, no one can become completely stress-proof. Even the Dalai Lama encounters stress. It is an inevitable part of life. Stress enters our life through work, family life, financial pressures, snarled metropolitan traffic, traumatic or troubling events, arguments with others, information overload in an interconnected world, and a hundred and one other flashpoints, or stressors. The fact that we will experience stress is inevitable and undeniable. Saying you will never incur stressful situations, or feel a little tense or uptight from time to time is like saying you will never see a teenager texting again. How we handle each situation spells out the difference between a life you embrace and experience fully every day, or one in which you cower in fear of the next stress-causing event.

A large amount of the stress you experience is likely to be completely unnecessary. If you learn the lesson that the stressful situation is presenting, you can become immune to those situations. You can deal with them without getting stressed. If you feel good about yourself, operate with high self-esteem and self-love, feel the love in everybody, everything and every moment, and approach each potentially stressful situation as a vigorous opportunity, you will practice a highly positive lifestyle where stress comes and goes–or even works *for you*. But how do you get from here to there? What if there was a way you could reduce your stress even more? What if you could become stress proof for at least half of your stress? What about 70%, 80%, or 90%?

Each of us is an individual with specific characteristics, personalities, tendencies and talents. We feel stress differently, and we deal with it in our own ways. We benefit in varying degrees from specific stress relief approaches. My hope for you is that the discussions, stories and steps in this book help you create a more effective blueprint for handling stress. With this book, you will be working from a template of proven solutions. While I can't promise that you will become immune to a specific percentage of future stress events or the stressors in your own life, I can promise that the steps in this book can help you minimize and/or alleviate most of the stress–and turn it around to your advantage. Many of my clients felt relief from *all* stress they were experiencing at that time in their lives through our appointments. The information in this chapter and book proved instrumental to their growth and success. A base result from these steps? At least 50% stress reduction.

By following the concepts in this book, clients have become happier. They notice the good things in their life, small and large, that they never noticed before. They overcome enormous traumas from their childhoods, past relationships, or even recent events. They appreciate the greatest joys of life–the little moments. Some of them never fully appreciated life until recently. Without stress, those little moments become magnified, more significant. My clients and others enjoy their friendships and family relationships a lot more. They feel more confident. They progress professionally in the workplace. They become more self-aware, noticing that the same things that bothered them before no longer aggravate them. They feel more capable of dealing with each and every situation, major or minor. When it comes to their interactions, they enjoy heightened awareness of the joys and worries of others. The old saying, "Walk a mile in another's shoes," becomes a working part of their daily life, not some ancient, bearded fable our grandparents passed down to us.

Let's embark on this wonderful journey. Like all worthwhile treks or voyages, it will be challenging at times, downright difficult at others. But in the end, we will work together to create a journey full of personal surprises. One that, I hope, will swing the doors wide open to the rest of your life.

A special gift for you:

I have created a website with special gifts to help you make the most of *DeStress to Success*. You'll find:

➢ Training modules to help you utilize the key stress reduction tools in *DeStress to Success*

➢ The *Am I Stressed?* checklist to help you find your true stress levels

➢ My *Stress Mapping Tool* to help you identify:

➢ the main areas of stress in your life

➢ where that stress is coming from

➢ your path to less stress

➢ Articles and resources to help you have more peace and enjoyment in life

To access these valuable gifts, visit
http://www.leowillcocks.com/bookgifts.html

Chapter 2: Seeing Both Sides

Serena Williams, Novak Djokovic and others feel it before their championship matches at the Australian Open. Performing artists get the jitters before taking the stage for major concerts or performances. Runners bounce up and down while lining up for their first marathons. Businessmen and women break into cold sweats before delivering important proposals or presentations. What they feel are the physical sensations attached to a single question: Can I do this at my best?

We hear stories all the time of people becoming sick to their stomach, sweating profusely, losing their appetites or talking at time warp speeds just before taking an important action–and delivering. They find themselves under enormous pressure to deliver and perform, and perform they do, often beyond what they considered to be their capabilities. When this happens, we applaud and congratulate them, ask for their "secrets," wonder how they rose up to meet such a challenge. And wonder how we can attain the same. Or if we can.

This ability to rise up to meet life's challenges exemplifies the positive side of stress. While we are socially conditioned to see stress as a negative–and, to be sure, this book has already underscored that point–stress is not an entirely negative condition. Not at all. It is *neutral*. When marshaled and channeled into something constructive and productive–a goal, the next job duty, your kids' education–stress serves as the driving force of keen performance. Stress often fuels your best efforts. I'd like to share a few simple, everyday examples of how stress works positively in our lives, and why it is just as important to keep our eyes on these positive characteristics as it is to minimize or eliminate the negative causes and effects:

o **People Perform Better Under Pressure**: I do it. So do most of you. It happens when we face a tight deadline or high-stakes task of some sort: preparing a presentation, getting products out on time, finishing a home remodel before winter weather sets in, and paying the tax bill. We stress over it, spend sleepless nights thinking about it, maybe we even snap at our loved ones over little remarks. Then we find a sixth gear, focus intently on the task, and get it done. Not only do we complete it, but at a level that outshines our normal performance. We take all the stress we feel, rechannel it into the job at hand, and convert it into a positive energy that drives us forward as if we were our own stampedes. We want to do our best, and our instincts and minds handle the stress. That said, we typically perform better under pressure in short spurts. Very few people can withstand the stress of constant, everyday pressure. That can be withering, and as such, unhealthy.

o **Some People Thrive in Competitive Conditions**: How many times have we seen people in the workplace, or on the athletic field, summon forth efforts and performances that leave us shaking our heads? While some people have trouble with the heightened pressure of competitive conditions, others thrive on it. They walk up to the proverbial starting line, and when the gun goes off, block out everything except reaching the finish line as quickly and successfully as possible. Do they feel less stress than the rest of us? Hardly; some feel more, especially when they're carrying the prospects of their office, home, company, or team on their shoulders. They worry, fret and wonder about their chances, feeling every bit of the discomfort and anxiety. However, when it comes time to hit a deadline, take an exam, finish the job or win the race, they funnel themselves into the moment, and turn stress into highly positive energy that drives their performance.

- o **Sex:** "Am I seeing this right?" you may be asking. "Did Leo just make a typo? How can sex be a form of stress? Isn't it, among other things, a form of stress relief?" Yes–and yes. Sex is our great expression of love, certainly a deeply pleasurable form of stress relief–and a stressful act. Only we don't think of it that way. We are so focused on the love, pleasure and satisfaction that we forget how many of our muscles are interacting with our limbs. Not to mention the stress on our cardiovascular system due to an elevated heartbeat and breathing respirations (as with other exercise). Why does sleep arrive so easily for us after we make love? Because our bodies are physically stressed–and need to rest.

In all of these examples, the important point to understand is that stress is neutral. It is neither positive nor negative, in and of itself. What we do with stress determines whether it will have a positive or negative impact on our lives. The natural reaction to a challenging circumstance is to see the negative impact it has on our lives - we all do this! But it creates unnecessary stress. As we move along, it is important that we learn to see the positives in every stressful situation–because, in many cases, what we perceive as negative stress may be a necessary, preparatory step to a very positive outcome. An example: burning the midnight oil, hands shaking, as you type out the final page of the proposal that ends up netting $100,000 in new business. When we learn to see this positive side to a challenging situation, our stress levels drop.

Life is full of opposites: positive and negative. Pain and pleasure. Comfort and discomfort. Love and hate. Emotions and experiences. How many times have those very emotions and experiences that once caused you agony, heartache and the feeling of failure ... generated growth, benefit and ultimate achievement or joy? So it can be with stress. Stressful situations actually benefit us, if we look at them more deeply. Think of a stressful situation in which you find yourself right now. Looks pretty challenging, doesn't it? Now let's flip the coin. This situation can be good, because it exposes the deep trauma that needs to be resolved. If we learn the lessons presented by our current stresses (and they all carry lessons), we can empower ourselves to achieve greater things and enjoy more happiness and success. It is through life's imperfections that we grow.

Let's return to the volcano illustration I presented in Chapter 1. When the resistance of gravity breaks, the volcanic magma explodes and releases the pressure from a century, two centuries... or forever. Even though this stress hurts, particularly when we feel like we're going to blow, think about what lies on the other side. If we can somehow overcome it, we can prevent pain in the future, and resolve bigger life challenges.

However, before we can transform our stress into a positive force in our lives, we often have to overcome what I refer to as "the Sob Story".

The Sob Story

If we hold onto our baggage, and dwell on it, we will likely develop a sob story, an excuse for not progressing in certain areas. This happens when we are bogged down in the frustration of what is happening, and we don't understand the positive effects of stress. Or, if we do have an intellectual understanding of it, we don't take the time and energy to make the effort. Even worse, we may actually believe that we can't progress because of that sob story. One man I know believes he has the mental capacity of a ten-year-old. So, he acts like a ten-year-old–a selfish one at that! He does not have friends, because he is selfish and takes people for granted. He expects others to be responsible for his actions and behavior. He can't hold down a job because he acts like an immature boy at work and causes trouble for himself and others, which leads his employers to fire him.

Realistically, he is very capable of progressing. He could easily act like an adult if he learned the lessons from his experiences, and moved the ensuing stress in a positive direction. He is capable of overcoming his baggage. It will require effort, and a new way of viewing the world and others–as an adult. He needs to choose to put his energy and focus into the actions that will help him move on. I have seen and helped people overcome much bigger demons.

If we are to work positively with stress, we must recognize the ways in which we bring stress upon ourselves. We cannot let our past and current traumas become sob stories. I can't think of many more debilitating ways to create and cave into our stress. It is important to be aware of why life presents us with certain challenges, so that we can better understand our current situations. We need to look at each challenge with the positive attitude of overcoming it. We gain from that which we face. Let us write this new story for ourselves. Make no more room for recurring sob stories.

As we review how different aspects of our childhood impact our lives as adults, it often comes down to our story, the tale we choose to tell others–and, more importantly, our inner selves. Acclaimed novelist Isabel Allende (*House of the Spirits*) once said, "Every time you tell your story, it is a different story." This is something we never think about when we share our memories, tales of woe or conquest, or personal love stories–but she is right. If you tell the same story, one day apart, you will certainly add a detail here or subtract a moment there. You may convey a different emotion. You might condense two old stories into one. Memory has a funny way of folding into itself, especially as we grow older. You may focus more on the challenge than the outcome–or vice versa. Or, if you grew emotionally or intellectually since the last time you told the story, you will present it with a different perspective or emphasis. Whatever the case, your story changes every time you tell it.

So why not focus on the positives? Why not focus on the positives of those stressful situations you managed to overcome? Why not show how stress worked for you?

Most of us are taught to focus on what is not good or right about our lives. We're taught to attract attention through our problems and dramas, a message that bombards us through advertisements, media and TV. Quick: when was the last time you saw a positive daytime drama? Or read good news on the front page of the *Sydney Morning Herald* or the *New York Times*?

This leads to my next point: social conditioning also contributes to sob stories. You might hear someone ask rhetorical questions like, "Why does this always have to happen to me?" "Why does it always go wrong?" "Why does Murphy's Law always have to be there?" or "Why can't things go right for me?" How many times have you heard those questions from others? How many times have *you* asked them–and then woven tales of woe and foreboding? If you take notice, many of the resulting comments focus on the worst of our lives. That's a sob story. The longer we hold on to these stories, the longer we hold ourselves back from achieving our goals. Our stories–meaning the stresses we've held on to, repeated, and may even define ourselves by– tend to hold us where we are. Why? Because they grow deep roots that expand into and draw from our tendencies, memories, experiences, dreams, relationships, loves, losses, triumphs, failures, and every other element that has clung to us since getting that first little whack across the bottom when we were born. The only thing more deeply rooted than stories in our bodies is our DNA.

If we can learn from and let go of that negative side of the story, and embrace the positive side, then we can let go of the stress and move on. There are always two sides to every story, no matter how dark or brilliant it seems at first glance. Understand that other side, and how it can benefit you. Also understand how the difficult challenges can benefit you, too, as you work to overcome them.

However, if we hold on to the sob story, and take center stage in the self-pity party, we will spiral downward. Everyone has stress and challenges. It is up to us whether we let it define us and become a sob story. Instead, use your story to spiral upward, to move on, to progress.

Two Sides to Every Life

The same childhood events that created lifelong baggage also helped to shape our personalities. They are part of what makes each of us a unique person. Understanding this helps dissolve stress that we feel about past events. It also gives us the opportunity to turn stressful situations into positive outcomes.

For example, one of my clients grew up in a family where her parents fought or argued constantly. Her childhood home was rife with contentiousness, and it was very hurtful to her at the time. Now, she is determined to enjoy an ever-growing, peaceful relationship with her husband. Every time they have a disagreement, they make the effort to resolve the matter peacefully. She works with her husband to keep their relationship alive and happy, and they operate with an open door to express their thoughts and opinions. They still argue now and then, but overall they have a very healthy relationship. She has taken her greatest pain from childhood and utilized it to fuel her greatest successes in adult life. Recognizing this positive effect of her childhood experiences enabled her to let go of the anger she felt about those experiences, and she now has far less stress. Hers is a wonderful, healthy perspective.

A different example comes from Charlene, who is being raised in a family where she is not the "golden child". Her sister, Mary, receives preferential treatment. Their parents usually settle things Mary's way, even if unfair to Charlene. Mary gets more chocolates and candy because Mary will sneak them out of the pantry and consume them before anyone else gets a single piece. Charlene often misses out. Meanwhile, Charlene is disciplined if she misbehaves, even if setting her own boundaries towards Mary. When Mary misbehaves, nothing happens. Charlene takes on more chores than Mary (who often doesn't do any; Charlene often finishes Mary's work, too) and is not appreciated for what she does.

Not surprisingly, all of this stress and mistreatment has created self-esteem issues for Charlene. She usually doesn't ask when she wants something. She has put off her own interests and desires because of the constant, almost certain disappointment of not receiving them. At the same time, she resents Mary and their parents. She feels very insecure about her place in the family. She gets upset when she misses out because of Mary getting her way. As Charlene grows into a teenager, she may look elsewhere for acceptance and love – not a bright prospect. She may accept relationships where her partner doesn't treat her with respect, just as she isn't treated with respect now. She may run through a series of boyfriends who cast her aside, when she only wants to please them. She will likely experience a lot of stress from what she is learning now – to allow others to overpower her, to subdue her own wants and needs.

However, Charlene is benefitting from her situation in a way she doesn't recognize. She is easy to get along with. Other adults enjoy her company, because she is so helpful and engaging. She plays nicely with other children, her kindness and caring nature appeals to others, and she makes friends easily. She does particularly well in school, and performs far above her grade level—one area where her parents properly recognize her. If she learns to love herself, set personal boundaries, voice her needs, and expect fairness from others, she will have good friendships and good relationships.

On the other hand, Mary is not such a pleasant girl. She swings between playing nicely with other children and being difficult and selfish. When her friends invite her over, their parents constantly have to watch to make sure she plays nicely. When she doesn't, she upsets the other children, but cares little about their feelings. Furthermore, Mary has to be urged to clean up after herself at other people's homes, and the parents eventually grow weary of her resistance and difficult personality. She is falling behind at school because her parents don't require her to do homework.

While at first glance, Mary seems to be enjoying the advantages of a spoiled childhood–treats, preferential treatment, no discipline, sliding on homework–she is missing out on important life lessons. Her apparent advantage is actually a disadvantage. Eventually, her actions will catch up to her, and she will have stressful events (like other children not wanting to play with her) until she learns to be fair, put in the effort, and be honest. She needs to take responsibility for herself and her actions, and to give a stronger effort in school and her other activities. Her lack of understanding over the consequences of her actions will serve her poorly in her adult life and create far more stress than a happier person will experience. In short, Mary is headed for challenges as she gets older.

Both Mary and Charlene are inherently good people. Unfortunately, the actions of their parents are impacting their psychology and beliefs about life. Charlene could learn the same good traits if her parents were fair, so long as they put in the conscious effort to teach them to her. While Charlene is being disadvantaged now, she is, in some ways, being given advantages as well.

I dealt with a situation that differed from Charlene and Mary's story in that the two sisters had serious conflict with each other. My client held serious resentment to her sister. As she put it, "What a controlling cow she is. Everything she does to me is trying to take control of me, trying to get me to live the way she wants, trying to get me to do everything her way. When I do something my way, it's never good enough, when I do something my way, she wants to change it. She wants me to change what I'm doing and when I'm doing it. Everything she does is to take things away from me." As we dialogued the problem, I guided her to recognize that there are two sides to every conflict, two sides to every story–and two sides to deal with it, one involving negatives, the other positives. Seeing the positive side would significantly reduce the anger and stress that she felt.

I asked her, "So how does this help you?"

"Are you listening to what I'm saying? It's not helping me!"

"Yes, I heard what you are saying, but I'm asking you, how does it help *you*?"

"You're not hearing me," she repeated. "It's not helping me, it's making me angry, it's frustrating me, and it's hurting me. I don't know what to do when I'm around her; I just don't want to be around her."

"OK," I said, "but how has what she has done or is doing … how has it helped you?"

"I don't know; it doesn't make sense. How could it be helping me?"

We dug more deeply. I explained that her big issue with her sister was that she was controlling, domineering, and didn't know when to stop. "Have you learned to rely on yourself?" I asked. "Because of your sister's behavior?"

"Yes."

"Have you learned to stand up for yourself?"

"Yes."

"Have you learned to do things the way you want, even if someone else doesn't want it done that way?"

"Yes."

"Have you learned to only take her opinion into account if it's going to help you to do what you want to do?"

"Yes."

Notice that, in this otherwise difficult situation, she answered four consecutive questions with "Yes." That flipped the coin of her dilemma onto the positive side. "OK, I've started you off, now you start. Where else is it serving you and helping you?" I asked.

"Oh, I've never realized that it's actually been a help to me."

We spoke for a while, during which she came up with a list of how her sister's actions actually helped her. She began to lighten up a little to her sister, then a little more. Finding these benefits was pivotal in the process of helping her let go of the anger and stress she felt. Eventually, she grew comfortable with being around her sister in a different role than a doormat.

By using this technique and others, the situation completely changed. She stood on her own two feet with presence of mind intact, even when her sister tried to do the things that used to annoy her. She felt confident within herself and saw that whenever her sister was acting like that, she became stronger by *not* allowing someone to push her buttons. And finally she felt free to live life on her terms, not fearing her sister's criticism!

Where We Find Comfort

Former Newcastle United football star Frank A. Clark famously said, "We find comfort among those who agree with us–growth among those who don't." This sums up life when we look at both sides of any situation. You can't have a negative without a positive. They exist side by side. Question is, which one do we see at the time? To which do we open our awareness in order to better see both sides, to see how it serves us? Or causes a problem? Once you learn from the negative, you can see its greater purpose and turn it into a positive. It becomes easier to love, or appreciate yourself, others and circumstances, whether you perceive them as good or bad. Chapter 4 has detailed steps on learning from the negative and embracing the positive in difficult situations.

When you see the positive, your perspective improves. You no longer are caught up in the frustration of the situation. You can recognize how any situation, no matter how difficult or stressful at the moment, is of benefit in the long run. This enables you to make better decisions. Your stress levels drop. You will feel better and at peace.

Victim? Or Victor?

All Jeanette ever wanted was for her two children to enjoy happy lives. She and her husband worked hard to provide them with a comfortable, although modest, childhood. They raised their kids outside the bustling metropolitan area in which they were born, moving to a bucolic country setting–twenty acres complete with horses, dogs, deer and woodlands. The plan was simple and sweet: work together, play together, raise the kids to adulthood while they were only in their late 40s, and then travel and enjoy a quiet, peaceful life with land and home paid off.

Then the walls came tumbling down. Jeanette's kids decided the country life was too slow and boring, so they turned to cheap thrills–drugs, teen sex, and drag races. By age 16, both kids were well known to the law for their misdemeanors. Jeanette kept bailing them out, holding tight to the dream she and her husband shared, and doing everything in her power to set her children straight … the way they were raised. The trouble continued. Warnings led to tickets. Tickets led to overnight stays in holding cells. That progressed into more serious offenses. The oldest child, Gina, became pregnant at 15 and had her third child at 20, and fully expected her parents to raise the kids so she could carry on. In the midst of this downward spiral, Jeanette's husband dropped dead of a heart attack at age 49.

Fast-forward ten years. Today, Jeanette raises three of her eight grandchildren, and keeps a close eye on the other five. Gina has spent three of the past five years behind bars. Jeanette's son, Steve, faces major health problems brought on by his own choices – and a tempestuous relationship with the mother of his five children. When their violent dust settled, he gained custody of all five kids. A year later, she disappeared entirely from their lives.

Jeanette was once a positive woman who loved everything about life, her eyes dancing with sparkle and possibility. Now, she blames her kids for everything she has lost and for all her suffering. She sees nothing good to live for. For years, she spoke of the beauty and presence of love and life. Today, she speaks critically, even harshly. This once beautiful woman looks thirty years older than she did ten years ago, and has lost all belief in the goodness of life. If you ever depict the long-term effects of hardcore stress, she would be the poster child. Jeanette has suffered terribly. She gave her kids a good childhood and constant love, and they "thanked" her by dumping their problems on her and constantly begging her to bail them out. As the loving mother, she bailed them out, every time she could. She feels like the victim–of life, her children, and even her husband for his dying so young.

Now for the tough question: who made her a victim? How would her life be different if she *didn't* bail out her kids in the beginning, but rather told them to pick themselves up? That she deserved to carry on with her life now that they were adults? Or, to do what she successfully did as a young adult–turn her challenges into a series of positives that otherwise could have been better appreciated by them?

It comes down to how we respond. Will we become the victim of that stress, of the actions of others? Or will we take positive actions and arise victorious over our environments and situations, no matter how difficult the challenge or intense the stress? Throughout each day, we wear different "hats", or take on different roles, depending on the task or situation. These hats may be father, mother, daughter, son, brother, sister, husband, wife, employee, employer, teacher (professionally or parentally), leader, listener, mentor, or caregiver. We play many different roles, of which two are most significant: victim or victor. We can be victims of our circumstances, like Jeanette, or create victory over challenging circumstances. Had Jeanette cared about her own happiness as much as that of her kids, she would have jumped off the runaway trains of their lives early on, before it became too late – helping them learn responsibility and doing everyone a favor in the process (and reducing her stress many times over). This is the nature of being a victor: not having power over others, but rather having personal power and strength. Obviously, Jeanette's children will still make their own choices, but the only way now for Jeanette to be a victor (and be happy) is to turn the situation around, and discover how the very things that hurt her the most are also helping her – to find positives in her current situation.

As Jeanette's story makes clear, it is important to understand how the people in your life will relate to you, and what they will expect from you. When you are around certain people, have you noticed that you feel insignificant, insecure, not as important, and not empowered within yourself? Or that when you are around others, you feel empowered, vibrant and strong, like things are going well for you?

I find two beliefs or thoughts frequently held by people in victim mode:

1. That there is not enough, things won't work, things are bad, or something is not possible to achieve or acquire

2. That they aren't good enough, things won't work for them, and it is impossible for things to turn around

They live with negative, discouraging beliefs about a certain situation. They have allowed life's twists and turns to deliver so many punches to their gut that they can't take any more–yet those punches keep coming. They can, and often do, direct their sad ways at the world: "It's too hard to get a good job, there aren't enough good jobs out there." Or, they turn it within themselves: "I'll never be able to get a better job; I'll never be good enough." This trips them up in many ways, wanting a:

good spouse, good employment, success in business, and financial wealth. Or, seeking respect from coworkers or people in general.

On the flip side, the victor believes:

1. There is enough, and things do work
2. He or she is good enough to receive or obtain what is being sought

Holding and practicing these beliefs goes hand in hand with being in control of your own life. When you feel this way, rather than being upset, or being controlled or manipulated in a difficult situation, you take control of yourself, set boundaries, and possess the personal power to change situations and circumstances for the better.

The problem and solution with the victim/victor mode constitutes flip sides of the same coin: "What you sow, you shall reap." If you think there is enough, and you are good enough for greater goodness to happen, it will–in increasing measure. If you think you're not good enough, and the world is piling up on you, it will–more and more every day. It's easy to fall into the *"poor me"* spiral. "Life is so hard," you might think, "why did they do that to me?" It's a true crawl-under-a-rock and hide mentality. Such feelings are evidence of a situation where we are not empowered, and carry resentment or other baggage. They are often a result of long term stress, as in Jeanette's case, but they also create more stress. This is why taking off the victim hat, and resolving the stress that has caused it, is so helpful.

Turning Around Difficult Family Circumstances

The story of another client illustrates this. She grew up under difficult circumstances. Her background wasn't rough, violent, or physically abusive, but things weren't emotionally stable. Now, many years later, she dreaded visiting with her parents. She intensely disliked speaking to them, even on the phone.

Furthermore, she wilted when viewing their status updates on Facebook, and their emails. Every time she contacted them, she fell again into this pit of despair. She felt that she was worth nothing, that she was insignificant and weak. Depression set in– every time. To say she carried a lot of unresolved baggage towards her parents is an understatement.

At the same time, she took out her feelings on her family and those close to her. She would treat her spouse and children the same way her parents treated her. She would speak down to them, become argumentative, and become abrupt and aggressive. She didn't want to lash out at her children, so she would avoid her parents, because she realized that only after seeing them did she lash out at her kids. Consequently, she would only contact them if absolutely necessary. When she did, she would try to think up ways of how she could stop them from overpowering her.

She didn't want to live this way. Who would? She wanted to enjoy her life. So we worked on these difficult issues, all of which produced negative stress, and helped her realize that she wasn't a little girl any more. It was time for her to grow up. She realized that she didn't have to be bossed around, she didn't have to be controlled or dominated. She was an adult and she could choose whether to keep being a victim – or become a victor. As the saying goes, she learned how to be "The Boss of ME." To help her, we created different activities to increase her assertiveness. She faced some of the horrors of her past. I helped her overcome her negative actions in each of those situations, so she could be more confident whenever they rolled around again (which they did). When she made the pivotal turn, she found ways to utilize the ensuing stress, and the situations themselves, for her benefit.

Today, when she contacts her parents, or sees their messages, she does not feel nervous, angry, hog-tied, or gutted. She remains within her own power and thinks properly on how to respond. She has released years of resentment while, at the same time, empowering herself with the new reality–her parents cannot dominate her anymore. She also has stopped lashing out at her kids. Her parents are still there, but her stress has gone.

This turnaround can happen in our relationships with a boss, colleague, neighbor or sibling. We can and do make a choice on how we let others impact us. Do we let the stress eat us up as victims–and pile on more damage? Or do we create positive results, take charge of our lives and become victors?

There are things that we cannot control, but we *can* control our self, thoughts, actions and emotions. We can control whether we fear things, people or events, and if we allow these things to control us. We may not choose some of the things that happen to us, or how others act toward us or around us. However, we all choose how we act or react. Even in hard situations, we have seen many victors emerge among the victimized. Why? Because they transformed the stress of terrible situations into positive outcomes, whether it meant repairing a damaged relationship, or trucking food into flood-stricken communities even after their own home was destroyed.

How do we better identify where we act as victims–and victors? And how do we transition from being a victim to a victor? One way is to find how the stressful circumstance actually helps us. With less stress and a better perspective, we can see the situation more clearly and act in ways to bring about better outcomes. I also have a series of questions I use with clients, based on the work of Dr. William Glasser, author of "Choice Theory"[1].

1. What is going on? Acknowledge what is going on. You cannot and will not fix it if you do not acknowledge there is a problem.

2. What do you want? Acknowledge what you really do want.

3. What steps and actions have you been taking to achieve what you want? What have you been doing? How long have you been doing it for?

4. How is your plan to achieve what you want working? Are you getting the desired results?

5. Are you willing to do something different? Think of the classic definition of insanity: to keep doing what you have been doing and expecting a different result. Are you open to exploring new ideas?

6. Ideally, what do you want to have happen? This is the same as the second question, except that I have added the word "ideally". In question two, you are opening to the fact that you are allowed to have something you want. Adding "ideally" can help you think further and deeper for what you want.

7. Which part of this are you in control of?

8. Ideally, who do you want to be in this situation? How do you want to feel in this situation?

9. If you were this ideal person, how would you feel? What would you think? And what would you be doing?

These questions helped me in my personal life. They also have helped my clients, and I trust they will help you further explore your sources of stress and your life.

Merry Go Round

Picture being a young child again, going to the fair, and riding the merry go round or carousel filled with toy horses; you wave to your parents or siblings as you pass by. You're having a great time riding up and down, waving to everyone, sticking one arm out, and enjoying the absolute freedom of the ride. Now fast-forward to the present. What if your life is like this merry go round, going round and round, with no end in sight? Not as much fun as riding carousels as a child, is it? Nor is it as carefree. In fact, the merry-go-round can consume your energy so completely that it leaves you with no strength or motivation to stop the machine, get off and walk forward.

In our adult lives, the same problems happen repeatedly, perhaps wearing different guises, until we learn their lessons. These start with unique challenges in areas where we might possess a character or physical weakness. They are so stressful because we don't know how to deal with them when they occur. If we can learn from these challenges, we can recognize and work to minimize or eliminate those stressors. They no longer become stressful to us.

However, what happens when we don't learn? When we choose to ignore or suppress a situation and the ensuing stress? The short answer? What I call "The Merry-Go-Round Effect". If you don't learn from your challenges, they keep reappearing in different forms. If you push a problem away, it will come back. Ten-fold. It will hit harder and faster than before, causing more disruption and stress. When it returns, and you don't work through it, the resulting stress will circulate throughout your life, spinning faster and faster until it overwhelms you and renders you powerless. For example, we might keep dating the same type of person because we are attracted to the same personality traits, including those that bother us. Or, we may repeat a many-year (or lifetime) cycle of recurring financial challenges over and over again.

The Merry-Go-Round effect must be overcome and redirected if you want to grow from the experience and have less stress. We can learn some of these lessons by gaining skills like money management or training in digital technology. With others, we need to go deeper into our upbringing or personality. Do we need to be more assertive? Calmer? More restrained? Stronger in tough situations? How do we determine if we need more training, or if we're on a merry go round at all? When you have particularly challenging, stressful situations, take a step or two back before responding. Ask yourself the following questions to identify your next moves:

- o   What is it I'm most bothered about?
- o   When has this happened before in my life?
- o   What lesson do I need to learn from this?

I find the Merry-Go-Round effect impacting clients in three areas above all others: relationships, work, and social life (friends, situations and experiences). Quite often, you'll find people in abusive relationships will bounce from one partner to another–or continue to take the punishment until they are broken shells of their former selves. The dynamics can include either an abusive male or female–or both–as well as physical, emotional, mental, and/or sexual abuse. There are many different types.

Now, what happens when someone finally musters up the courage to say, "I'm not going to put up with this anymore, I'm leaving," and they leave? Then they find a new person who's wonderful and caring, everything they ever wanted? Only to discover, that after a period of time, this person's true colors appear and he or she ends up being almost identical to the one they left–or escaped–from.

Wow, what a merry-go-round! Sadly, they've encountered the same problem with a different face. A couple of features might have changed, but not the end result: they find themselves in physical or emotional peril. Thankfully, many domestic violence shelters provide counselling to help sufferers regain confidence and self-respect. These services, and others, have enabled many to step off the merry-go-round of abuse, and embrace happy lives and healthy relationships.

Have you noticed that, if you are submissive or easy to please, or feel like you may not deserve the best, that people possessing the traits that give you difficulty keep appearing? It's like the person who quits drinking because he cannot stand being around drunk people, or cannot stand his own tipsy ways–and then, years later, must confront a raving alcoholic who ruins his otherwise enjoyable outing at an outdoor concert. There are physically abusive, domineering, possessive, angry, back stabbing, controlling, untrustworthy and manipulative people everywhere. As long as we don't know how to deal with that type of person or situation, or the stress that comes with it, and until we gain the confidence, self worth and understanding within ourselves to *know we deserve better*, we will keep the gates open to allow these people into our lives.

A client of mine had been emotionally abused for a long time. One day, she finally drew the courage to leave her husband, after which they divorced. Since then, both she and her ex-husband have remarried. She married a man who seemed different in many respects, but later proved to be similar in personality to her ex. A year later, they separated. She couldn't understand why. Likewise, the ex-husband married someone similar to his ex-wife. The only real difference: one has blonde hair, and the other is a brunette. Apart from that, they were nearly identical in personality, mannerisms, and the way they addressed others. So weary was my client that she summed it up by telling me, "All men are the same."

That's a statement from someone stuck on the merry-go-round, spinning inside her negative opinions and experiences, far from the truth. All men are quite different from one another. There are common personality traits and similarities, but not all men are the same. Nor, for that matter, are all women. Only when we become so myopic and lose perspective do we feel or believe this way. And nothing destroys perspective like an abusive relationship.

Yet, there is also great truth in her statement *as it applies to her current station*. Why are all her men "the same"? Because that is what she is unknowingly attracted to! Why is she attracted and vulnerable to that type? Why does she like specific traits or features? Because she wants to be needed. She's on the merry-go-round of being needed! She's comfortable with it, and then she gets annoyed when her man turns out to be more of the same. Her compulsion to feel needed draws her to men with major problems, often narcissistic or even sociopathic men who needed looking after, whether physically or emotionally. At first, it felt great to her, and why not? She was *needed*. When she burnt out from lavishing constant attention and energy on the man, however, the man's deeper problems would surface–a daunting task for any woman to deal with properly.

Until we deal with our baggage, and confront and overcome unnecessary beliefs such as "all men are useless", these issues will crop up. When the merry-go-round spins faster, the collateral damage will become greater. A quiet disagreement becomes a loud argument with very cutting words. A slap on the face becomes a punch in the ribs. A comment to "quit looking at men that way" becomes a direct order to never communicate with a man. A request to spend less time on Facebook becomes a cutting off of the Internet and a cell phone disconnection. This is not childhood. These merry-go-rounds are not fun.

And that's just relationships. What about the work carousel? A quick story: a client of mine was a sales representative, very good at his job, and earning big dollars. Then, suddenly, he was not being paid for his work. No matter how many customers he brought into the company, he was not adequately reimbursed. The papers were lost, or something had happened, and these customers had apparently decided not to go forward. Such were the excuses from "above". Later, my client discovered that some members of higher management were stealing sales from him, claiming they had negotiated and closed the deals themselves. Subsequently, they drew the ongoing commissions from his hard work. He tried to sort it out, but eventually grew so angry that he left the company without confronting the others.

He found a new company and started over. He worked hard, got into a good sales rhythm, pulled in nice commissions that added up to a considerable income, and added lots of new clients to the company's portfolio. Then the same thing happened. He only received some of the commissions to which he was entitled. They started "losing his paperwork". He started asking, "Why does this keep happening to me?" His stress mounted. My client was stuck on an accelerating merry-go-round. He was vulnerable to the same sort of people who engaged in the same predatory and manipulative business practices. The only difference? The faces and company names. This happened at four or five different companies. He couldn't understand why it kept recurring.

I asked him to remember the first time he could recall someone treating him disrespectfully, being dishonest, and stealing from him. The first time turned out not to be a professional situation at all. It actually involved his mother. When he was a child, his mother told people that she was happy giving birth to her son and raising him. Within the family however, it was well known that he was not wanted. She never really cared for him. She didn't feed him properly. His mother always gave him the smallest servings at dinner of any child, regardless of his appetite. He had to buy dinner each night after eating at home. He didn't have a bedroom–his bed was in the laundry. Her daily mannerisms, and the way she spoke to him, made it clear he wasn't loved. She even told him that he was not wanted. She said the only reason he existed was because his father wanted another child.

When his mother told others that she was happy with him, he thought her dishonest. He felt disrespected in the way she treated him. In his mind, his mother stole his childhood and withheld the nurturing, unconditional love that a child is entitled to receive from their own mother. Likewise, at the time of our appointments, he felt that the companies were stealing from him–stealing income which he used for his physical nurturing.

Once we spoke about this, I used questioning techniques to help him discover how the events with his mother were actually a service to him. How did those things benefit him? How did they help him grow, and become the person that he is today? What good did they do for him?

The benefits included:

- He learned to become independent and self-reliant. This helped him to develop professional drive. He didn't want to be dependent on others, and he was willing to handle any and all tasks himself. As a result, he performed well in sales. He was a good, honest salesperson. He learned how to relate to people, and his customers liked him.
- He learned not to assume that all people were kind and caring, and to take people for who they really were.
- He realized that in picking a spouse, he wanted someone who would care for children. His choice of spouse had the potential to have the biggest impact on his life happiness. He found someone who would be the loving mother to their children, and had a lot of joy from that.

When he saw the benefits of his relationship with his mother, much of the resentment and frustration disappeared. He felt less stressed about the past, and able to move on. He felt confident that when he looked for new work in sales, he would find people who would treat him respectfully, be honest, and pay him fairly. He no longer needed that lesson any more. He had learnt from it and grown from it. Within weeks, he took a new sales job with a company that started out paying him fairly. Years later, they still pay him what he's earned. Through the process, my client realized that if he didn't learn a lesson in one area, he would have to learn it in another. He wasn't reliving it in his family life, but professionally.

Now let's look at the association between the merry-go-round and friendships. For my first few years of high school, I attended a specific school. I had some good friends, and we all thrived from a shared cultural diversity. My friends included a few Pacific Islanders, Middle Easterners, Europeans, and Aussies– both white and indigenous. The mixture of personalities was equally rich, but we all got on and we all had fun. Together, we played basketball and many other sports. We had strong friendships.

Then I moved. I attended a new school. I was excited about the change, but upset to be losing my friends. When I arrived, I made some new friends, but I also realized I was the only Anglo Saxon among my new group of friends. Every other person was Asian of some sort, mostly Filipino, but other oriental nationalities as well. It didn't matter to me–or to them. There were similar personalities to those in my old group of friends. We forged strong friendships.

Point is, the merry-go-round doesn't have to be bad. Know that when it is bad, there is a solid reason for it. Work hard to understand the reason so you can switch to a better circuit. Make it work to your advantage. How to do this? It takes action, and the right activities. Deal with what is happening now, and the original cause itself. Explore it, dissect it, face it, and deal with it. You will become empowered within yourself by learning to deal with negative situations as they happen. Convert each situation and its accompanying stress into a positive solution–and enjoy the positive side of stress.

I'd like to end this chapter with an instructive story on the ravaging effects of unchecked anger – and how we can turn that around. Rebecca was a middle-aged woman under great stress in many areas of her life. We started working on helping her with her self-confidence so she could move to where she wanted to see herself. Throughout the process, I did not know that she had wanted to leave her husband. She never hinted at it until she told me she had left him. I knew they were having issues, but she certainly never suggested it was bad enough to leave. She told me that she had wanted to leave for quite some time, but never thought she could. She feared what people would think of her, and what he would do to her. This all came back to her confidence, a big part of the reason why I was counseling her.

Confidence did not come easy for Rebecca. For years, it didn't come at all. When Rebecca was three, her grandfather started to molest her. When her father found out, instead of protecting her, he decided to tag team with his father-in-law. Five years later, both her grandfather and father had a problem with gambling. To pay off some of those debts, they pimped her out. If she did not perform, she was beaten and then forced to perform anyway. Her father would take photos of her acts with a Polaroid camera, so that their clients could have a lasting memory of their experience (all part of the service).

When she was in her mid-teens, Rebecca's grandfather tried to have his way with her again. This time, her body stopped him. The more he tried, the more her body shut down. He grew so enraged that he picked her up and threw her into the cupboard. Rebecca quickly picked up her clothes and ran out. As she was leaving the room, he said to her that she was now good for nothing.

Throughout this time, Rebecca had no one in her life to talk about the molestation. Her much older sister always had an excuse for not being home. When Rebecca would bring it up to her mother, her mother would either not listen or give her the wooden spoon. Both of her grandmothers had passed away. She suffered in silence until she ran away.

The impact on Rebecca as an adult was predictable: she felt powerless and worthless. She never felt confident to voice her opinion or needs. When she married, her husband treated her disrespectfully. While never hurting her physically, he was domineering, possessive and selfish. Whenever she tried to communicate her needs, he always dismissed her and spun it back to what he wanted. She always felt insignificant, and that she was never good enough as a mother. When she found out that her own daughter was raped, and when she had high suspicions of her children being molested, she blamed herself. She felt that she was a total failure as a mother. However, Rebecca was a great mother. She supported her children through their ordeals to the best of her ability. She spent time with her children, cared about them, and still exudes that genuine love for people.

When Rebecca came to me, she said that the only reason she felt she was still alive was to fulfill men's sexual desires. Even then, she still felt violated and dirty. She also had a benign growth on her thyroid. She was scared, because her only option, it seemed, was to undergo thyroid removal surgery, which she didn't want. This growth was so large that breathing and talking became more difficult. Not to mention that the thyroid's dual roles, to manage energy use and dictate metabolism, were thrown out of whack. As we discussed the thyroid's role, we tried to ascertain the relationship between her stress and healthy weight.

Many people with thyroid problems also stress about their weight. We found that, in Rebeca's case, her stress was due to the fact that the growth was squashing her voice and suffocating her gradually. We talked about why she felt unable to voice her needs, and where that had happened in the past. That's when her horrible story of being abused emerged.

Through all of her ordeals, Rebecca never felt she could voice her opinion or needs. Her abusers would not let her. Now the thyroid growth was physically stopping her. The growth was actually a trigger to help surface the pain from which she had hidden for years. After discussing the emotional connection between her past and the thyroid growth, I knew one tool that would help her overcome the pain from her experiences: to recognize the hidden benefits of her incredibly challenging experiences.

Whoa. That's what she thought, too. At first. She needed to see how all of those traumatic, terrible experiences had actually benefited her. I explained to her that every event has good and bad points. Even the most challenging experiences have benefits. In fact, our biggest pains can empower us for our biggest successes.

Not only did she need to understand this in concept, but also to see how it had actually happened in her life. We started looking for benefits. It was not easy, but once she got started, she actually found them. She saw that she was understanding of others in similar situations. She was a great support to her kids when they had similar problems. When she was abused, she had no one to talk to, and always thought everything was her fault. She didn't want her children to feel the same, so when they were abused, she helped them to open up. They were able to free themselves of the pain of it a lot faster.

She kept her close relationship with them, unlike her mother. Rebecca wanted nothing to do with her. This was actually a benefit to her, because she never felt she needed her mother's approval when making decisions or living her life. She was free to live her own life without any bearing from her mother's expectations and opinions.

Another benefit she discovered was that her challenges helped her desire faith. Her upbringing was not religious at all. Most people reject new ideas and habits because they hold on to what they grew up with. Because her past was so painful, she was willing to do something different. She found a church she liked; it brought peace to her life. Through the years and challenges since then, her faith has kept her life steady. She has meaning and purpose. Her unconditional friends support her through her healing processes. To a degree, she even loved herself–most significant, considering her upbringing.

I also gave Rebecca activities to build her self-confidence. She had a lot of success with these (they are covered in Chapters 4 and 8). Today, she sees the amazing person she is. She is happier. She looks younger and healthier. She feels happy within herself. The growth on her thyroid has physically shrunk. It doesn't stop her from breathing or talking properly anymore. She is confident. And, when she needs something or has an opinion, she voices it! She has finally overcome the pain that held her back for so many years.

Her process of overcoming her trauma, and the overwhelming anger it created, has helped her accept the things she can't change. She now knows she can't change her past, and isn't trying to hide from it any more. She has also gained the courage to change what she can change – her life, on a daily basis. And she feels she has the wisdom to know the difference.

She gained the courage to walk away from an abusive husband. Normally, I work with clients to overcome the problems they are experiencing and overcome the need for a divorce. But if abuse happens, take care of yourself. Right now. No matter what. As Rebecca saw things clearly in her life through our appointments, it confirmed that she had made the right choice in leaving him. She had the courage–no small task.

Out of all of my clients, Rebecca has worked the hardest between appointments. Because of her effort in the activities I gave her, and the techniques we used, she experienced this incredible turnaround in *four* visits.

Chapter 3: Stress and the Natural Relationship Cycle

Even on the best of days, relationships create challenges and opportunities. No other aspects of our lives seem to demand more of our attention, presence, communication skills (verbal and non verbal alike) or expertise in relating with others. As often as both parties are in sync with one another, emotionally and verbally, one or the other can also operate on a different wave length. That's where the challenging questions start to pop up: What can I say (or do) that will alleviate the concern? Do I understand him/her correctly? How can we use tonight to be closer? How can I better serve my partner?

These are questions for good, stress-free days, for relationships rolling along smoothly without undue or outside interference. What happens when we inject everyday stress into intimate or family relationships? What happens when concerns appear like: job or financial pressures, the need to relocate, communication breakdowns, growing incompatibility, or kids whose problems drive the parents apart? What happens when, like pit bulls clamping onto a poor animal's neck, they hold on and won't let go?

The answers–or non-answers–to these questions lead to very busy therapists' offices. Everywhere you turn, people are focused on relationship issues. Experts, hosts and guests talk about it on daytime TV. Bookstores are filled with magazines and books pertaining to relationships. We catch the latest relationship-oriented movies at the cinema expecting some sort of clash or conflict, and waiting for the resolution. What would the motion picture industry be without relationship problems–both on the silver screen and real life?

I feel that a principal, fundamental cause of relationship difficulties is overlooked, even ignored at times: the part stress plays in weakening and sometimes breaking the relationship bond. Also, how one of the biggest sources of stress comes from within family relationships. Even the healthiest marriages experience stress from time to time. Have you ever attended a Silver or Golden wedding anniversary party? Sometimes, you'd swear the guests of honor are as relieved to have made it through 25 or 50 years as they are ecstatic to be sharing the celebration with the ones they love. No relationship is immune from day to day stress. Even the best relationships go through cycles of stress and challenge, along with the more preferable cycles of fun, enjoyment, and peace.

When we don't know how to deal with the challenge that stress presents, our relationships can turn destructive, create more conflict, and potentially lead to separation or divorce. When this vicious cycle spins, it sucks all of our love and dreams into it. We feel like we're plunging into a black hole–one that sometimes takes years to recover from. Some don't recover at all. How did the person we love madly become our enemy? How did those endless, fun and loving conversations devolve into two people who can barely say "hello" to each other? How did life's challenges and stresses mix into the Molotov cocktail that blew up your once great relationship?

It doesn't have to be that way. Once we learn how to deal with these challenges, we can resolve stresses as they arise. We can also nip the problem before it starts to eat away at the foundation of our relationships, or marriages, built with years of our lives. We can grow from our stressful experiences and form a stronger relationship through the challenges we overcome. In the next couple of chapters, I will discuss several sources of stress and tension in relationships, and how to deal with them appropriately. My primary goal here, as it is with my clients, is to replace misunderstanding, resentment and pain with trust, appreciation and respect. This discussion can help you immensely in your intimate relationship. Most of the information works well in all of your relationships with others–children, parents, colleagues, and friends.

The Natural Cycles of Relationships

All long-term relationships pass through different cycles. They include: the excitement of a new relationship (the honeymoon period), challenging times often further exacerbated by undue stress and power struggles between parties, working together and a feeling of deep appreciation and gratitude after the challenges are resolved. In this latter stage, one partner looks at the other and thinks: *How did I ever live without this person? I can't imagine a day without them.*

These cycles, or stages, are essential for the growth of the relationship and each person within it. Through them, we find our way to communicate (even our little phrases in our own private language, spoken between each other, a sure sign of intimacy!), deal with problems together, and handle the stresses that will surely challenge us from outside forces or the relationship itself.

It's important to realize this. Otherwise, you may compare life now (possibly a challenging time) to how it was when you first met (probably the most enjoyable). If you think things like "he used to be so much more romantic" or "she never used to tell me what to do", then you are comparing the present moment with the past. Let's face it: if you're in a relationship of more than three or four years, you can easily revisit those first weeks or months, sprinkle some fairy dust on them, and find yourself in a glorious kingdom of carefree love. Looking back on it, you will probably feel something is wrong with your relationship today. You will also perform a disservice to yourself, because we always overly glamourize the beginnings of relationships–and we can never go back to the precise date and circumstances that sparked our first moments together. What we can do, though, is bring forward the essence of that magic. It will generate what we truly seek at our core: ever-deepening love and happiness.

The Honeymoon Period: At first, the honeymoon (or new relationship period), seems the best. After all, it is the most fun. This new person in our lives excites us. We might have met under everyday circumstances, or our love might have kindled on a beach in Tahiti. No matter *what* the location or opening moments, they were emotionally supercharged. We never forget this feeling. Those prone to commitment use the feeling as a vehicle to deepen their love. Those who aren't commitment-oriented keep trying to re-create the moment, which can lead to trouble.

In the honeymoon period, we thoroughly enjoy doing things and spending time together. We see many good traits in our partner, without concern for weaknesses. We're made for each other. Every day is a good day. We may even count down the days or hours until we see our lover again. Because we have not been together long, we have not pushed each other's buttons. We hold a lot of trust for our partner, because we know they would do nothing to hurt us. Ever. This is a time of closeness. We wear rose-colored glasses–and see only the rosy side of things.

What fun! What love! What togetherness! Hold that feeling. Treasure it. Enjoy it. However, realize that the honeymoon period will only last so long, from several months to a year or two (if you're fortunate). Eventually, the rose-colored glasses will come off. When they do, the challenges will begin–not a bad thing. Not at all.

The Balloon Popping Period: What happens when the air has been let out of your big, happy relationship balloon? Challenges start to surface. At first, you might be surprised. After all, your agreeable partner starts to disagree with you, and conflict rushes out of the joy. How did this happen? *Weren't we blissfully in love, relishing life in our private little cocoon just last week?*

At this point, you begin to experience the challenges described in this book. Your disagreements may be caused by misunderstandings in the way men and women communicate. The actions of your partner might push your buttons and bring up baggage from your past. You feel hurt, shocked and upset, not just because of what they did to hurt you, but because they hurt you at all.

If you understand that relationships take work, you will find it easier to deal with this period. If you really connected and *communicated* well with your partner during the honeymoon period, this phase will be easier. It will also flow more smoothly if you choose a partner who handles conflict calmly and is willing to compromise–and listen.

Ultimately, the way to deal with the balloon-popping period is to resolve each problem as it arises. Don't put it off until tomorrow, no matter what the problem is. If conflict arises from any of a thousand possible sources, and fires up more than once or twice, find the true cause of the conflict and resolve it. Quickly.

Let me share an example. Thomas, a client of mine, received a major shock when the balloon first popped in his relationship. His fiancée, Elsie, almost ended their relationship over their *first* real challenge. Their relationship had moved along smoothly and strongly for a while. Thomas regularly took romantic actions such as buying flowers, decorating Elsie's car with paper love hearts, showering his affection through numerous calls and texts, and even creating short holidays for them whenever possible.

However, as their wedding drew closer, they spent more time organizing the celebration. This activity was far different than any others in their relationship. Under the best of circumstances, weddings aren't the easiest things to plan. As the stresses of the wedding grew, Thomas and Elsie found it seeping into their relationship. Eventually, it sparked their first major conflict. In the ensuing argument, Elsie reacted loudly and verbally. When it became more heated, Thomas took a drive to calm down, so that he wouldn't say or do anything to make the problem worse.

No such luck. Things got worse. Elsie phoned him and said she couldn't possibly marry a man who was going to run away, who wouldn't stay and fight his way out of a conflict. She preferred that he stay and argue, rather than step away to calm down. At this juncture, she was willing to leave him over this single argument!

As I worked with Elsie and Thomas, the real problem became obvious. Whether or not Thomas realized it, Elsie's buttons were being pushed. Elsie associated Thomas' decision to leave in mid-argument with her father's choice to leave home–permanently–when she was a girl. Thomas' departure brought up Elsie's feelings of abandonment, insecurity, and pain–none of which pertained to her fiancé. She didn't want to risk going through the hurt of losing someone close again. For that reason, she almost ended the relationship.

Elsie wanted Thomas to stay and fight–the very thing that, ironically, often causes relationships to break down and one of the parties to leave for far longer than a one-hour cool-off. Why did Elsie prefer this approach? Because she watched her parents argue it out, toe to toe. After many years of arguing, their relationship deteriorated. When her father finally stopped fighting back, he left. So Elsie associated Thomas' decision to disengage, to *not* fight, with leaving and insecurity. She associated fighting with security–because her father stayed home when he fought.

During a very long conversation, I helped Elsie recognize why she was so upset with Thomas' decision to leave. I also helped her see that arguing, in part, caused her father to leave. It wore him down to a point that he didn't think his marriage was worth salvaging. She eventually realized that Thomas' choice to leave and calm down, then return home without further delay, was a good thing. He was making sure he didn't say or do anything to cause more pain. He was protecting her, himself, and their relationship.

Elsie saw how much Thomas really loved her. She began to feel secure when Thomas drove away, or went to another room, to avoid a conflict. She also began to see that her way of handling stressful or challenging events – through verbal explosions – did not benefit their relationship. This story has a happy ending … or might I say, a happy unfoldment into their ongoing lives. Thomas and Elsie got married, and are still married to this day. They still deal with challenges, like all committed couples, and see me every now and then when things get difficult. But they have grown so much together in their relationship. Their love for each other has grown markedly. They handle their challenges and conflicts more appropriately. As they face and overcome baggage from their past, the same deep issue that caused conflict before – namely, Elsie's Dad leaving his family behind – doesn't create friction now. They understand each other and enjoy many good times. They are more confident, independent and happy than when they first met.

Day-to-Day Rhythm: After the bubble bursts, a new period begins: the day-to-day rhythm of life together. Both people experience the challenges and joys of day-to-day life. You get to know each other more closely while recognizing and learning to live with the good and bad qualities of your partner.

If you have a long-term relationship, you will spend a lot of time in this phase. It's simply called *life*. It offers plenty of enjoyment and challenges, both of which you will experience many times. For this phase to move smoothly and steadily forward, the most important action you can take is to resolve challenges as they happen and not allow them to ferment into long-term issues. Some challenges will resolve themselves, quickly and completely, but the majority will need appropriate attention. Unfortunately, complicated relationship issues are not as simple as that first big kiss we gave each other.

During this time, regularly expressing gratitude and showing appreciation for each other is essential. Without it, you can easily forget about all the good points of your partner. Everything from work to daily responsibilities can muddy the waters in which you once saw your partner's face as though it were reflecting from an alpine lake. Keep your eyes on that reflection; hold on to the beauty of your partner.

Be sure to communicate clearly. Sharing common goals, such as staying married/together your entire lives, raising a happy family or making sure your retirement plans are in alignment, is vitally important. Reaffirm your commitment to each other. There are other measures you can take to keep your relationship alive, which we'll discuss later in this section.

Keep your relationship healthy so that it can survive the rocky periods. They arise from challenges within the relationship, extended family troubles, financial issues, etc. Challenges might be difficult, but every time you overcome them, you strengthen your relationship. You grow as individuals and a couple. You learn to remove baggage and pain from your past. Remember that. It helps to alleviate the stress that seems to swirl into any difficulty.

Deep Appreciation and Love: One day, years into the relationship, you wake up, look over at your partner, and either say or think: "I feel more love for you than I ever have before." Even though you don't feel all the electricity and excitement of the honeymoon period, you actually feel closer, and deeper. When challenges arise, you feel that your partner is your best friend, the one person you want at your side as you work through the situation or issue. When the good times roll, who better to share them with than the person who's been at your side the whole time?

It takes some couples 50 years to get to this point, while others reach it in five or 10 years. The time period is not significant. What is, though, is how it feels to reach this place.

Your heart and soul will feel golden. You will feel so attuned to your partner or spouse that the world feels like your playground, and the most outlandish dreams or figments of your imagination feel readily attainable. However, once there, you won't necessarily stay there. You may enjoy this almost supernatural connection for a while, but then you may find yourself back in the day-to-day rhythm period as you face new challenges and conflict. When those issues are resolved, the feeling of deepest appreciation and love returns. Therein lies the beauty of reaching this stage: it keeps returning as long as you address challenges as they arise, and continue to build your relationship.

Appreciation is the king, queen and royal court of the successful relationship. Gratitude and appreciation are two of the secret ingredients in that awesome meal shared at your favorite romantic restaurant–the meal that tastes much better than when you cook it at home. The third secret ingredient? Love. Love always deepens when you add gratitude and appreciation. Gratitude is the ultimate antidote to resentment.

Unless you make an effort to seek out and call attention to the highest qualities and most generous actions of your partner, you may fall into the trap of seeing only their downside when daily stresses hit. This happens with both men and women, though more with women. A biochemical process called Female Stress Syndrome triggers in their brain, fueled by releases of Epinephrine (adrenaline) and Cortisol, the "flight or fight" hormones, that prompt them to instantly remember the bad things their man has done–even if those incidents took place ten years before! This was perfectly referenced, with dry humor attached, in the 2005 film *Two for the Money,* starring Matthew McConaughey, Al Pacino and Rene Russo. As they walked down a New York City street, and Pacino's character was openly thinking about drinking again, Russo's character said, "Walter, don't go there. That's a bad neighborhood for you." Later, she said, "Don't take me up to the second floor," meaning, *the floor in my brain where all the bad things about you are catalogued.*

Another problem is that you may forget to thank or show appreciation for your loved one. This particularly happens with men, who sometimes think that because they have thanked their partner once, she will carry that gesture far into the future. That's not how it works. Women need to be thanked and appreciated repeatedly. If not, when they get stressed, they start to remember the bad actions, and forget how much appreciation, care, admiration or respect their partner showed previously. If allowed to fester, these situations can build an unhappy relationship.

When you show gratitude and appreciation, both you and your partner benefit. When you receive the grateful action (being thanked), you are happy for being appreciated and admired. You feel valued. As a result, you are more inclined and willing to help in future situations. If your partner thanks you and shows appreciation consistently, you will feel the joy of extending kindnesses of your own accord–or increase what you are already doing. Likewise, when you give and express gratitude, you feel happier and more loving because you have noticed the good your partner has done for you. You recognize and focus on the good in your partner more often. As your partner becomes more willing to help (because they feel valued and wanted), you become even more grateful and appreciative. Soon, your relationship strengthens. You still frustrate each other sometimes, but not nearly as often. When you feel stressed, you now feel *happy* to have your partner, happy they stand by your side. They are part of the solution, rather than the problem.

How to Show Gratitude

- Thank your partner when they do something kind for you
- Thank your partner when they do an everyday thing that contributes to the relationship (dishes, mowing the lawn, etc.)

- Make an effort to notice at least three good things about your partner each day. Compliment them by sharing the three characteristics, traits or qualities. Appreciate them not only for what they do, but also for who they are. An example: "You are so patient with the children/grandchildren. Thank you for being so patient."
- Women: when a man does something kind for you, tell him that you admire how well/thorough/fast he does it, as well as thanking him. Compliment him on the job he's done. An example: "The lawn looks so neat and tidy now that you've mowed it. Thank you."
- Give notes of appreciation and admiration
- Thank your partner every day and compliment them every day–both on what they do, and who they are.

In some ways, gratitude is similar to giving. This is because giving gratitude, appreciation and admiration is a type of giving. It is a very essential way to give in a healthy relationship.

The Ways We Handle Stress

Men and women handle stress in different ways. Seems obvious, doesn't it? You'd be surprised at how often conflict erupts because we *don't* notice this difference. While we naturally (and correctly) assume that every person handles stress in their own way, it is vital to understand–especially for the sake of relationships–that men and women are biochemically and emotionally wired to handle stress *differently*. How many times have we asked ourselves or others, "Why can't he deal with stress as well as I do and talk to someone about it?" Or, "Why can't she just let it go and move on instead of going over and over and over it? Why can't she just let me figure it out for myself?"

In a sense, these questions are unfair–especially if the improved health of your relationship is your goal. Here's why.

When stressed, women generally talk to others and get support. They talk out the problem and move into solution mode. On the other hand, men prefer to think it out. They might go out to the shed or garden, exercise, or find another form of recreation or emotional outlet to help them forget the problem for the time being.

When a man withdraws, the woman likely will sense it. Unless she has learned otherwise, her first reaction is worry. She may consider his withdrawing to be unhappiness with her, and seek reassurance by talking to him. This will bother him more; he wants time to himself. He may even snap at her. Ironically, her inclination to reassure and nurture, a maternal instinct, will create the exact opposite of what she intended.

Consequently, his sense of withdrawal may leave her feeling neglected or uncared for. She may not even realize he is stressed. Why? Because *he hasn't told her*. In her eyes, he has withdrawn without explanation, and she feels raw because of it. Feelings of neglect from her past may surface. There's that merry-go-round!

Women and men can help resolve any stress caused by this situation. First, they can realize *how* they handle stress differently. When men start to withdraw, they can reassure their partners by saying, "I love you, sweetheart. I'm just a little stressed right now, and I'm going to take a break. I'll be back soon." When a man communicates in this clear, simple manner, it is important for the woman to not dig harder to root out the cause of his stress. If she doesn't already know, then she's best off not asking. Pumping him with questions is definitely a no-no. She needs to trust him to figure it out for himself.

If the onset of stress and the man's emotional withdrawal happens at a time when a woman really needs her partner's help, at that moment (such as brewing mayhem with a child or teenager), she can say "OK, take a moment, but I really need your help. Would you help me as soon as you are able?"

When an otherwise emotionally available man withdraws from a stress-related situation, he needs time to process. Once he has resolved the stress, and calmed his mind and heart, he will return and be more loving. Men can help the cause by returning with complete focus and attention for the partner's needs. This will help reassure the woman that everything will be OK the next time he needs to withdraw.

On the other hand, when a woman talks about her problem, which usually happens when something starts to bother her, misunderstandings can arise. Men sometimes mistakenly feel that their partners are blaming them. They may think their partners are unhappy because of the circumstances of the problem; they imagine their loved ones saying, with a finger in their faces, "it's your fault; you are duty-bound to have prevented it." For this reason, men can become defensive and react when their partner is upset.

Another potential problem occurs when a man tries to fix the problem that causes the upset. Or, worse, what he *perceives* to be the problem. Being a man, he's going to perceive now and ask questions later. He may tell her how to fix the problem, and what to do about it. He's helping her, right? Wrong: it only makes the situation worse. As he moves into solution mode for the most superficial part of the problem, she feels he doesn't care about her because he isn't listening to her–or her heart.

The third potential problem comes when a man tries to help his partner feel better by explaining to her why she doesn't need to be upset. Once again, he is trying to help, but instead worsening the situation. A not uncommon response from a woman in this scenario: "Since when did you know and understand everything I'm feeling right now?" When you hear that, back up. You have stepped too far.

Men and women can work to prevent conflict in any stressful situation that can lead to these problems. For a man, the most important action is to listen, and remember that she is not blaming him. When a man listens to his loved one without suggesting "answers" to her worries, she knows that he really cares. She feels important when he listens. She knows he really loves her. He honors her presence in his life. For that central reason, it is important that her partner actively listens when she is feeling upset. How do you do this? By maintaining regular eye contact, and making listening sounds when appropriate ("mmm", "uh-huh", "yes I see what you mean"). If a man can answer any follow-up question the woman asks, then he's listening. Also, he will show how actively he listens by avoiding all distractions, not working on anything else simultaneously, and exercising tunnel vision for the length of the conversation.

When the woman feels cared for and able to freely talk about the problem, she will usually get out all of her frustration. She will feel better, and a potentially more stressful situation will be diffused. Women can help by reassuring their partner that they love them, believe in them, and are not blaming them. They can make an effort to not use blaming words, because in some cases, they might actually blame their partner. This is all part of remaining in control. Expressing emotions and engaging in yelling matches create two far different outcomes. The more women and men stay in control, the more their partners will listen and respond positively.

How would a healthy venting conversation start out? I would suggest she say something like this to begin: "I'm not blaming you, thank you for listening"; or "It's not your fault, and thank you so much for listening." When she is finished, she can thank her partner again. It is very important to say something like: "Thank you for listening, I feel so much better now." With this action, the woman shows how much her partner has helped and supported her by listening. It goes against male instinct–we want to act, solve, fix, mitigate or eliminate the problem (plus, we have all the answers, right?),–but it *works* when diffusing stressful situations in relationships. The next time, when her need to express so many thoughts without getting an answer bewilders him, he will remember that listening is the best way to help.

Men and women are meant to be different. While we obviously share many things in common, our differences can sometimes cause problems in relationships. I don't mean differences in our likes and dislikes, but rather, those fundamental differences in how we think, feel, act, and handle stress. When we don't take the time or effort to understand this in our partner, we set ourselves on a course of misunderstandings and hurt. This can happen even when we have the best intentions! Few things pump stress into an otherwise calm relationship like misunderstandings and hurtful actions.

We cover many differences in the ensuing chapters, but I would like to point out one in particular that can upset the natural cycles of relationship like no other: the need for the man to be trusted, and the woman to feel supported.

Men Need Trust, Women Need Support

Trust is the center of a man's universe. His sense of self-worth and purpose revolves around trust. He wants everyone to trust him–especially his spouse or partner. When she trusts him, he feels "good enough," no matter what else is occupying his life.

Interestingly, the issue of trust lies at the root of why men often are resistant when a woman offers advice. When a woman tries to help this way, she approaches from the kindness of her heart 99 percent of the time. However, the man often (mis)interprets it as a message that she doesn't trust the way he would handle, or is handling, the situation or issue. *She doesn't trust me,* he might think.

This also explains why men generally don't offer help when women perform physical tasks. Even if you obviously need help, if you don't ask, they trust you to get the job done. From a man's perspective, it's a sign of respect. Problem is, women don't know that this non-offering of help is a compliment. They feel hard done by. When a man wants help, he will ask. That is why it is fine for a woman not to give advice; he will ask if he needs or wants it. Give him trust instead.

On the other hand, women want to feel supported, cared about–and cared for. While it is OK for women to not offer a man help (or advice), the man's best course of action is the opposite: to offer her some help. It means you really care about her and really love her. Likewise, if you don't help, she may feel that you don't love her. This is why women give so much advice. From their point of view, they are helping.

Once we recognize and understand these differences, we can better picture how conflict arises so easily. A woman offers or gives her advice as a gesture of love, to which a man grows defensive. Feelings of not being trusted in his past surface, worsening the problem. However, if he understands his partner is giving love in her own way, he can accept her offer graciously, even if he chooses not to utilize her advice. Either way, he handles it better. If his partner then understands that advice is best given sparingly, when requested, he will feel a lot happier.

Men also love to be admired for their ability to perform tasks, functions or noble actions. A woman can help a man feel more needed, admired and trusted by complimenting him for his performance in specific tasks. The more she compliments, the more valued he feels, so long as her praise is genuine. She also builds trust in her man by refraining from correcting him when he makes a mistake. She trusts him to figure it out himself. Moving one step further, a woman can ask his opinion of the best option when faced with an important decision. If he replies with "It's up to you", she has received the ultimate nod of trust from her partner. It's a win-win.

A woman feels hurt when she perceives her man "not being there for her". If he doesn't offer help and support to resolve a situation, or an emotional difficulty, she may feel unloved. She may grow upset from her perception that he doesn't help. In her mind, he doesn't care anymore. If she understands his choice not to help is a sign of trust, and she remembers to ask for help when she needs it, things will run more smoothly.

Women love to see devotion in their men. A man can help a woman feel more loved by prioritizing time with her. He can help her with many tasks, especially when she seems tired or unable to start or finish them. It is not an insult to offer help to a woman; it is the quality of a truly noble, devoted and loving man!

Chapter 4: How Relationships Generate Stress

Imagine a beautiful wedding in a lush, green garden. The bride stands before the witnesses in a beautiful, elegant dress. Her gushing groom holds both of her hands while adorned in a sharp, expensive suit. They look deeply into each other's eyes as the minister reads out the wedding vows. Finally, he turns to the bride and asks:

"Do you take this man to be your lawfully wedded husband, knowing you can walk away at any time?"

To which the bride replies, "I do", her eyes gleaming, her dream has come true.

The minister then turns to the groom. "Do you take this woman to be your lawfully wedded wife, knowing you can walk away at any time?"

"I do," the groom says.

While this example seems humorous, almost farcical (it came from a "no lock in contract" pay TV ad), it serves as a sad reality for many. Most people don't enter a marriage or a relationship thinking they can walk away at any time. We want it to work out. But at the same time, if someone hurts us deeply, and keeps hurting us for a sustained period of time, then our best options might be separation, break up or divorce.

Welcome to many of today's relationships. What we see in the wedding scenario is the "before" frame from a movie we'll call "How Relationships Generate Stress". The paragraph preceding this one is the "after" frame, the final scene, the one we once imagined filled with sunsets and palm trees, but instead turns as dark and haunted as the aftermath of an Alfred Hitchcock or *Batman* movie.

While most people acknowledge the impact of stress on their relationships, far fewer understand how relationships generate stress in reaction to those outside pressures–or completely on their own. Imagine two different pictures. One is a room encased in see-through, bulletproof glass. Inside, you see two people, clearly in love, smiling and holding each other. Outside, objects bombard the glass, from rocks, darts, and sharp objects to sonic blasts. It's as though the couple is hurtling through the asteroid belt! Yet, they remain solid, together, undeterred by the maelstrom.

Now for the other picture. Two people stand in an room filled with glass windows, peering out at their dreams: vacation getaways, outings with friends, beach after beach filled with perfect waves, bookshelves overflowing with titles they've never read, concert dates for every band or orchestra they wanted to see, their adult children's newly purchased homes. They see the glorious, hard-earned ticket to their golden years. Inside the room, however, it feels like the business end of a typhoon. Husband and wife tear at each other, flinging emotions and barbs like wind-whipped waves, pummeling each others' hearts and eroding everything good they see in each other. With each new stress the outside world hurls at them, the tempest intensifies. Finally, it blows away their dreams, love, trust, and friendship. For either to regain peace and order in their lives, someone has to move on.

That's what ingrown stress does to relationships. My goal is to help you identify those internal causes from within your relationship and show you how to work with them so you can dissipate and eliminate them. Once you can do that, no outside stress will be strong enough to bring down your relationship. You will be surrounded by an emotionally bulletproof shield. You might take a hit or two, but it won't knock you out.

However, if you increase stress within your relationship dynamic, then *every* outside stressor that pops up will push your emotional buttons. When that happens, you will find yourself in a very difficult situation, where relationship survival is endangered.

Let's address some key causes or actions behind ingrown stress.

Dealing With Our Non-Commitment Culture When Committed

When faced with challenges in your relationship, you can act on one of three options. Most people only acknowledge two. I'm sure that you have heard these statements, just as I have: "It's better to leave someone than stay in a relationship where you are fighting and you're not happy"; or "It's better for the children if you leave each other than stay together and fight all the time."

Only two options are being acknowledged: divorce or separation, and staying together while miserable. It calls to mind the tongue-in-cheek wedding scenario I painted at the head of this chapter: in many ways, our culture offers a way out from the moment we say "I do." This non-commitment culture, as I call it, truly is first generation stuff. Our Baby Boomer parents or contemporaries married with a lifelong intention, but many divorced as society became more open to the idea. Many of their children, of whom many are in their 20s to 40s, grew up in single-person households with non-committal parents. It became *normal* to many of them to be products of a divorced family. As for previous generations, they knew nothing of the sort. Divorce was only an option in the most extreme situations. When you look at it socioeconomically, women didn't have a real choice before the 1970s; until then, there were very few well-paying jobs with which a single female could raise her family. Many women remained in marriages for this reason as well.

In many ways, we're pioneers on a scary journey. In the United States, 53 percent of marriages end in divorce. The numbers aren't much different in other countries; for instance, Canada's rate stands at 48 percent, the UK's is 47 percent, and Australia weighs in at 43 percent[2].

Now that I've changed your dreams of marriage to a nightmare, scaring those dreams of marriage right out of your head (for which I do apologize), what about the third option? The one to which many of our parents, and nearly all of our parents' parents, yoked themselves? The "til death do us part" option? It might just always be the most enjoyable option, that's for sure.

The problem is, in the middle of a crisis (or after years of feeling unloved), we don't feel that option three is possible. We don't even feel it ever existed–at least not for us. When entombed in these moments of despair, it feels like nothing will work. Now, imagine the stress that creates when your partner *is* a third-option person, one who feels a lifetime commitment is exactly that. Or, imagine the stress between you and your partner when you can't see your way out of a problem, and make a decision to part ways–only to have the heavens unload on you in the form of judging parents, society, friends and your own expectations. Either way, enormous stress brews between the two of you, making the situation appear dire.

But option three is still there! With the right advice, many relationships can be helped. If both people want to work on the problem, check egos and judgments at the door and seek a solution, then there is a *strong* chance of regaining your loving relationship. You have to put your commitment above all else. Many relationships pass through rocky periods and emerge stronger because of that commitment to try to work it out, no matter what. The one exception: physically and/or long-term emotionally abusive relationships. If you are caught in one, then move on. Option three is not for you.

I know an American couple that came together and had an incredible relationship–until she began demanding to know where he was at all times. He gave her no reason to feel that way, despite his somewhat frequent business trips. Accustomed to living on his own terms, he eventually buckled from her demands and *did* give her a reason; a few weeks after breaking up with her, he temporarily took up with an old girlfriend.

After three months of being separated but mutually miserable, despite dating others, the couple reunited. They entered counseling, where two fears surfaced: the man's fear of being 'tied down,' locked into a commitment after two unsuccessful marriages; and the woman's fear of being cheated on, which her ex-husband of 20-plus years created through countless dalliances with other women. Yet, this couple loved each other very deeply, a love bolstered by a friendship as deep as a fairy tale–they'd been friends for almost fifty years, since playing together in *kindergarten!* When the depth of their love and the mutual trust of their friendship aligned, they again grabbed onto the third option. Their fears disappeared. He loves the commitment to a lifelong relationship, and strengthening it every day. He begins by letting her know his daily plans. Now, she supports his hectic schedule without questioning him–at all. The ingrown stress that fractured their relationship no longer exists. It is gone. They built the bulletproof glass around themselves, and they deal with external stressors directly and appropriately. These two fell in love after vowing they would never commit to anyone else. Now, they've created a solid commitment for the rest of their lives.

If you have a long-term goal for your relationship, such as staying married/together your entire lives, and do what it takes, you will more than likely ride out the storms. Act to bolster your goal as well. Build love by taking the actions that make your relationship happier–giving, appreciating, compromising.

Think of a relationship as you might think of educating yourself: the learning never stops. There is always something new, something fresh. Learn how to communicate and have a loving and enjoyable relationship. Iron out the problems along the way. Overcome the fears and stresses from your past when they surface. As I said in Chapter 2, if you don't handle them, you may find yourself in relationships that repeat the same problems, because you never learned how to deal with them.

If you already have a mountain of relationship issues, don't give up. Start today. Work on one issue at a time. Every time you handle an issue, you will reduce some of the stress while simultaneously strengthening your commitment and sense of resolving problems together. After each issue is resolved, celebrate a little! Go out for dinner. Take in a movie. Sit on a park bench, or walk on the beach. Reaffirm your love and devotion to each other. Turn that old tendency to de-commit into deeper commitment. Do what you can to keep it alive!

Where's the Stress Coming From? A Present Situation? Or the Unresolved Past?

Relationships face a lot of hurdles. They include time pressures, not enough time together, misunderstandings, different priorities, financial challenges, selfish behaviors, and unmet expectations. This list could wrap around a major city if we all threw in our contributions. However, one challenge has little to do with your current relationship. Rather, it reflects more on your past.

Let's go back to the couple in America. They entered their relationship with everything on their side: a lifelong friendship, well-rounded experience, high levels of fitness and health for their ages, strong careers, common friends, and common interests in cycling, running and bodysurfing ... I could go on. Yet, each possessed one major hurt from the past that almost killed their love–his fear of commitment, and her fear of infidelity. Nothing in their present lives was capable of derailing their relationship. But their past experiences nearly did.

In a relationship, situations will pop up that instantly hook into your past, like it or not–much like the merry-go-round we discussed earlier. When that happens, we experience feelings from that trauma that have been bottled up for years, or decades. We often react inappropriately in the moment, because we are trying to respond to the present situation but are being driven by unseen forces from our past. We think our pain arises entirely from the current situation. Once we recognize that our present stresses and stressors often funnel from past sources (like the volcano to which I alluded in Chapter 1) we can handle present situations more peacefully.

My client, Janet, offers a perfect example of this. When Janet was a young child, she was serially molested. Her mother remarried several times, and each of her stepfathers molested her. Janet grew up in silence, continually being molested by each male that came into her life. Once Janet became older, the molesting stopped. However, its impact on her life continued.

After reaching adulthood, Janet found a kind, caring man and married him. He was nothing like the men that molested her, but her past still caused trouble for their relationship. When they would retire to the bedroom and begin to make love, everything would progress smoothly and enjoyably until Janet would suddenly shutdown completely and become disinterested. She would not allow their lovemaking to progress any further.

This proved very challenging for her husband. He thought there was something wrong with him, something she didn't like, but out of respect or concern for his feelings, wouldn't tell him. Many men could develop quite a complex about this and even get defensive: "Why won't she share herself with me?" "Aren't I good enough?" "What am I doing that she doesn't like?" and he might even get defensive.

However, Janet married well: her husband was a patient man. When she explained what had happened to her as a child, he found it quite challenging, but sensible. Over time, as Janet faced the horrors of her past, and they worked together on it, she overcame her past experiences and they went on to enjoy a healthy relationship–in all ways.

Another example of past-infects-present comes from conflict. When a conflict arises, the ensuing stress seems out of proportion with the severity of the original problem. Often, it is. Here's why: the current event, conflict, issue or action reminds you of similar past situations that didn't end well. Consequently, your past feelings of distrust, frustration, violation, or anger surface to hit the current situation like a sucker punch, out of (apparently) nowhere. The current situation is blown out of proportion, and an ensuing anger response follows that is often hurtful–and completely unnecessary.

Physiologically, your brain recognizes the past stressful situation as a threat. When something even remotely similar to that situation happens, your brain automatically shoots out the cavalry of cortisol and adrenalin: you're on red-flag, DefCon 5, fight-or-flight alert. Brain activity lowers in your prefrontal cortex (your logic center) while your limbic system–the emotion and survival center–is primed for battle. Your brain prepares you to act *now* without a conscious recognition of all past threats. You lock into the situation that has triggered your survival response–the current event.

This type of response is supremely challenging in the emotionally charged dynamics of relationship. More than likely, you already know this. Women, when your partner doesn't engage you in conversation right after walking through the door after a hard day at work, how do you feel? And how do you feel if *you've* had the hard day, but he doesn't engage right away? If you're accustomed to it, then you may give him some time to unwind before sharing your day with him. If not, his apparent insensitivity might kick up old pain of parents not listening to you as a child, or your previous boyfriend never listening when you were upset. All of that past hurt comes roaring back. Maybe your partner just needs some time alone to unwind so he can throw himself 100 percent into your world emotionally. That way, he will care more about your feelings and listen attentively.

In any event, the likely reality is that he loves you and cares for you immensely. He may just need that little bit of time to unwind, shed the skin of his work day–and, perhaps, the fires he had to put out amongst his colleagues–and then bring you his best listening ear. But that's not how it feels at that moment!

Now to the men. Let's be honest: don't you find it frustrating when your spouse continually asks you questions about your day? "Why doesn't she trust me?" you might think. However, once again, your anger stems from more than your spouse's well-meaning, love-first questions. Did someone distrust you in the past? Did your mother constantly tell you what to do and "help you", not giving you the chance to fend for yourself? Did past girlfriends ask questions constantly, tell you what to do, or simply not trust you?

That's what happens when our past comes roaring back. It creates stress that never belonged there in the first place. When one person or the other doesn't realize or know the past connections, then serious damage can–and often does–ensue.

How do we decipher all of this so we know which conflicts are fed by the past–and which are completely created by a present action? Here are a few questions that I run through with my clients that are very helpful:

- When has something like this happened to me in the past?
- What happened then? Did it turn out well?
- Could some of my anger/frustration/hurt and emotional reaction result from that situation?
- Is this current situation really as bad as it feels?
- What can I do to better handle this situation now?

You can think more clearly about the current problem by asking these questions. You may not need to take any action at all. The situation may be nowhere near as bad as it seemed. Or, you may take action. Either way, you will have recognized the underlying reason for a lot of your stress, and separated it from the present situation. That gives you a much better chance of resolving the problem instead of adding to it.

The Price of Judging and Daring to Compare

Have you ever thought that your partner wasn't good enough at something? Not romantic enough? Athletic enough? Smart enough? Or stable enough financially? Did you wish they would show more understanding, less bossiness, household work ethics to match their drive at the office, or more decisiveness?

When was the last time you thought this way? My guess: more recently than you might admit. Join the crowd, we're all in the same boat at times. When you last thought this way, did you consider why you wanted your partner to come up to your desired speed in that certain area?

Why do you want your partner to act differently? What are your reasons? See if any of these ring familiar:

a. To attain a certain result: cleaner house, more money, more romance, less arguing, etc.

b. You know someone much better in that specific area, quality or character trait than your partner, and wish your partner was more like them (whether a real person or fictitious character)

c. a + b

More often than not, the answer at first seems like a. But with more thought, and some self-reflection, you realize it is almost always c: a + b. Most people want a result they seek, but they also compare their spouse or partner to someone who seems more successful, better skilled or more sensitive in that area. Past or present.

When we compare one person's strength to another person's weakness, we judge the person with the weakness to be unsatisfactory, or somehow worse. At the same time, we esteem the person with the perceived strength to be superior. Imagine the stress that places on our partners when they are the subjects of our comparisons–and yet, we compare more frequently then we might imagine. You may have already been a little dissatisfied with your partner in that area, but the comparing and judging only amplify your feelings beyond what is appropriate for the current situation. This often results in emotional responses that are hurtful and build resentment. Plus, the chances of you getting the change you want diminish even further.

When we compare people like this, we miss the full picture. We miss it big-time. The person we judge harshly owns plenty of strengths and weaknesses, but we only acknowledge *one* weakness. The person we esteem highly possesses strengths and weaknesses, but we focus entirely on *one* strength. When we judge and compare, we fail to appreciate our partners for the generally well-rounded, loving and caring person they are. Instead, we feel dissatisfied, shortchanged, or even resentful. We ignore all of our partner's other strengths–no doubt, there are many. While we only may think about it for a few minutes, our dissatisfaction toward our partner can affect the way we feel about our relationship. Ladies and gentlemen, this is a primary source of paralyzing stress created from within the relationship– and one of the most preventable.

One of my clients, Mia, experienced firsthand the relationship challenges of one partner judging the other. Her husband, Nicolas, demanded a spotless house. Mia obliged: the floors, windows, windowsills, counters, ceilings, were almost always clean. The cupboards and bedrooms were organized. The laundry was washed, folded and put away like clockwork. The dishes were always washed, dried and stacked in the cupboard. The wood was polished regularly. Mia even mowed the lawn, weeded, and kept the outside of the home tidy – jobs that typically fall on the man's side in many relationships.

The constant work tired Mia. She didn't like always cleaning their large house, in part because it prevented her from spending time with their young children. Despite Mia's great effort, Nicolas remained unhappy with her performance. He would often compare her to his mother, with no shortage of verbal chidings or even abuse. Apparently, in his mother's house, you could have eaten dinner off the floor. He routinely ignored Mia's strengths to focus on what he perceived as her one weakness.

Tension ensued. She grew resentful of his insatiable demands, and he remained dissatisfied with her. On top of that, the children started to disconnect with their father. The more Nicolas spoke rudely to Mia, the less they wanted to be around him.

Eventually, Mia stopped cleaning so much and spent more time with their children. The house was still kept clean, just not spotless. And occasionally, Nicolas came home to small messes. You can predict what happened next: he became more rude and angry. Mia felt he didn't care about her, and stopped trying to live up to his expectations. The children grew more upset with their dad. The relationship continued to spiral downward, all because of Nicolas comparing his mother's greatest perceived strength to his wife's one perceived weakness.

During our work together, I met Mia's mother-in-law. I asked her what she thought of the situation. She said that Nicolas did not remember that when he was younger, their house had its fair share of messes. Only when he and his sibling grew older, she told me, could she keep the clean house that *she* coveted. No one, such as a husband, pushed her. On top of that, Nicolas' mother had only two children. Mia and Nicolas had five–all under eight years of age. Keeping a home spotless with five young children is not an easy task, even for a superhuman!

Nicolas failed to see the big picture. He was comparing Mia to an illusion. In his mind, his mother kept the house clean while looking after the kids. She could clean better; Mia could not clean well enough. He laid unrealistic expectations on his wife. The illusion, which created his problem, was that the house was always clean. In reality, his mother never kept the house clean until her two children had grown up.

Nicolas was completely aware of how he compared Mia with his mother. But this isn't always the case. Often when these thoughts bubble up, you feel unhappy with your partner, but don't realize you are comparing them with someone else. Only when you stop and think about your actions, and the dissension and unhappiness it is causing your partner and yourself, can you see it.

When you find yourself dissatisfied with your partner, take these steps to help you identify the person to whom you are comparing them, why you are making the comparison, and the illusion possibly moving through your mind:

1. When did I start feeling this way about my partner?
2. What brought my partner's weakness to my attention? Was it the action of someone else with a strength in this area?
3. Who has a strength in this area that my partner is lacking? (It could be parents, siblings, co-workers, friends, partners of friends and co-workers.)
4. Once you have identified the person or people, take note of how you are comparing your partner's weakness with their strength. Recognize that your partner has many strengths, and the other person has many weaknesses.
5. Create a list of 20 strengths you see in your partner. Remind yourself of these strengths whenever you start to focus on a perceived weakness.

6. Look at both sides of the equation. What are the *benefits* of your partner having this weakness? What would be the *downside* to your partner possessing the strength to which you are making comparisons?

7. Final question: Am I comparing my partner to an illusion?

I can't stress the importance of Step 6 enough. It is how you resolve dissatisfaction and resentment if you are judging your partner.

In Nicolas' case, the downside of Mia keeping the house spotless proved to be a major issue: she couldn't look after the kids properly. They would fight amongst themselves because they weren't getting any attention, very unpleasant for Mia, as well as for Nicolas when he got home. They would also break things and make even more mess while playing unsupervised for long periods of time. Because of this, Mia was missing out on her children's childhood–one of the elemental joys of being a parent. This added to her misery and stress. When Nicolas came home from work, an exhausted Mia resented him. Their relationship lost all of its enjoyment. Bedroom time was almost non-existent. So she stepped up. She decided to partake in the lives of her kids. They became happier and fought less with their mother giving them more attention. If Nicolas didn't react to the mess when he got home, they were happier to see him, too.

However, this was just one of several relationship challenges. Since Nicolas didn't want to work on them, he and Mia eventually divorced. My role with Mia shifted to helping her through the stress of the divorce, as well as Nicolas' increasingly vindictive behavior after they separated. I helped her deal with the stress of legal proceedings, custody issues, and his nasty phone calls, so she could be strong for herself and her children. Mia came through this challenging time and exerted the confidence to make tough decisions that were best for herself and her children. Consequently, she is a happier, stronger and more independent woman, and has gained a lot of self-respect, which took some effort after all the years of being mistreated. Meanwhile, Nicolas finds himself on the merry-go-round of failed relationships. He never learned to appreciate his partners, always comparing them with his mother.

Once you look at the pros and cons your desired trait brings to the relationship, or the benefits and downsides, you will resolve a lot of dissatisfaction with your partner. By honoring each others' strengths and respecting each other's weaknesses, you will also strengthen your bond and reduce the stress. You will look at each situation more objectively, and see if you hold unrealistic expectations toward your partner. You can decide if you really want your spouse to change in that area–or let them carry on. If you do want change, ask politely and directly as opposed to creating a conflict. Prefacing any such request with "I love you, because of ….", and then bringing up the matter, goes a long way. There is more detail on how to peacefully ask for your requests later in this chapter and in Chapter 5.

Judging happens in both directions. When a woman gets flowers at work from her partner, but her colleagues do not, then those ladies might go home and stick their partners in the bad books for not delivering flowers to *them* recently. Conclusion: they aren't romantic enough. This does happen.

One place of inevitable comparison, a real danger zone, is the bedroom. Many of my female clients share relationship issues that stem from being pressured to do things in the bedroom that do not sit well with them. They feel compared to past relationships, and/or the things men see in pornographic videos, movies, and magazines. They want to share their love and express themselves in one way, but the partner expects something totally different, out of their comfort zone. Many of their partners view porn, thinking this is normal, what everyone is doing. (Though not as prevalent as men, even a few women do it, which can make men uncomfortable as well). They neglect to realize that porn stars are *actors*. Partners confuse fantasy or made-up scenarios with reality. Porno movies are *movies*! Though they may seem real, they are completely edited.

My clients feel violated because of the acts they are compelled to perform. They want to be themselves, to share their sexuality in their unique way. After all, isn't sexuality between loving partners supposed to be about *love* and sharing between one another? This situation causes unnecessary tension, and a level of stress beyond belief. It ruins relationships.

Hannah and James

Hannah was frequently upset with James because he was not working enough in her eyes. She wanted to achieve their financial goals faster, and she wanted him to work harder to accomplish that. Hannah would let James know by venting at him for more than an hour, repeatedly. However, these were more than simple venting sessions. Hannah would directly accuse James of not working hard enough, frustrating him. He felt belittled, not trusted or admired, and would react. Sometimes, he could keep his cool, but the internal frustration and tension were building within.

James had moved states to be with Hannah. He opted out of the final year of his college education, and basically had to start afresh. He was in a menial part time job with reasonable pay, a stepping-stone while he decided what to do with his career. This didn't feel stable enough for Hannah. Ironically, what brought them together (his moving from one state to another) triggered the problem.

Hannah directly compared James to her parents. Even when her family had all the necessities, plus extras, investments, and were financially secure, her mother constantly pushed her father to work more and more. Her mother wasn't polite or even negotiable about it, either. She would berate and criticize Hannah's father, telling him he needed to work more so they could achieve the next financial goal faster. As a result, the man held three jobs for a long time. Hannah felt secure in this; it was all she had ever known.

Hannah wanted James to exhibit the same level of commitment to financial goals as her father. When he didn't (couldn't) do so, she grew frustrated. She was mirroring the actions her mother took. Only one problem: James was not Hannah's father. He wasn't as easily "persuaded", for one thing. Even if he was, he couldn't do what she wanted.

Economically, times were not as good for James as they were for Hannah's father. This was the post GFC economy. He had moved states. On top of that, Hannah was expecting James to achieve in a few years what took her father decades to build. She was comparing James to an illusion.

When I saw Hannah, she openly talked about how James could not do what her father did well. However, she didn't realize that her feelings were influenced by her comparison. I helped her to see that not only was she comparing them cognitively, she was comparing them emotionally. By idolizing and esteeming her father's financial success, she was creating dissatisfaction with James, *no matter how well he performed*. She also was ignoring James' many other strengths.

Awareness was our first step. The second was to see the positive qualities of James, and the drawbacks of her father's actions. She was only viewing the good side of her father and the bad side of James. She needed to see both sides of each. I asked her to tell me downside of her father working so much, and her mother's demands for financial growth. At first, she couldn't do it. Then I asked her, "How often did you see your dad? How much did you get to spend time with him?" She replied that she hardly ever saw him. She never got to spend time with him at all, aside from when he disciplined her.

"How often did you do family activities?"

"Hardly at all."

"Did you go on family vacations?"

"No."

I pointed out that her mother and father put financial growth as their top priority. Unfortunately, it rose so far above the rest of their lives that everything else suffered. I helped her realize that her parents didn't have a good relationship. They didn't have much time together because her father was working so much. When he was home, they didn't get along well, partially because of the way Hannah's mother spoke to him – the way Hannah was now speaking to James. Everything was work, work, and more work, with no time to play.

"Is this really what you want for your relationship with James?" I asked Hannah. She replied that she didn't. Through our process, she saw that her parents' imbalanced pursuit of financial growth was not completely good. It had its drawbacks. It was destructive for their family.

I then helped her to see the good in James. I asked whether James spent any time with her. What was their relationship like when he was home? Would that be different if he worked three jobs? Did they go on vacations together? Would they be able to have a close relationship if James lived up to the comparison she built? Hannah realized that James was very different to her father, in ways she liked. In fact, she loved these differences most about him. If he did work three jobs, she would not get to see that part of him. When they were not arguing (about their financial goals), and he wasn't stressed about it, James was romantic and committed. He valued their relationship highly and spent time with her. He took responsibility for chores around the house. Family time and a healthy relationship were important to him. He worked, but he didn't want to work so much that he'd never see Hannah.

Once Hannah saw how she could not have both sides of James at the same time, she realized that it wouldn't be great after all if James worked three jobs. She realized that they were still on track to their financial goals, and she could be happy to let the process take time. They had accumulated savings, which were steadily growing. She stopped harassing James. She saw the good in him again and was happy with him. She no longer expected him to be like her father. James was relieved to have peace in the relationship again. He was able to release his frustration, and their relationship again became enjoyable.

A few months after overcoming this hurdle, James found a training job in a well paying trade. He is still on training income, but when fully qualified, he will be earning an above average income while working just one job. They won't progress at lightning speed financially, but they will balance financial growth with a great relationship.

Always Avoid Assumptions

What happens when we judge and compare too much? Besides stirring up far too much stress and bad feeling, we often fall into the habit of making assumptions. We assume the other person's intentions, their likes and dislikes, or how they're going to respond. Or, we tell them how they feel, how they *ought to* feel, or why we *know* they will act in a disagreeable (to us) way.

Assumptions happen not only in committed relationships, but also with any interpersonal contact. It commonly occurs when we feel stressed. Assuming the worst of someone is often a reaction to a stressful situation–one that piles additional stress onto an already smoldering moment or day. An example of this comes from my own life. Sometimes, I work late from home. At the same time, my wife gets our children ready for bed. I emerge from my office, well after their bed time, and see the kids still up. I would say, "Why aren't they in bed yet?" or "It's way past their bedtime, what is taking so long?" Predictably, she would (justifiably) reply with, "Well, you could help."

Looking back, I would be frustrated by the time I walked out of my office, because the children weren't in bed. I didn't want the children to be tired and grumpy the next day–a direct result of staying up too late. In the moment, however, I didn't think about why I was stressed. I just thought my wife was taking her time to annoy me. I was making an assumption about her intentions. At the same time, I was also judging my wife. I was comparing my best to her worst, in terms of the time it would take me to get them into bed. Or, even more to the point, what time I would choose to put them down for the night.

When I thought about it, I realized that getting the children to bed fast was not the only goal. I noticed that sometimes when I got them to bed quickly, they were not happy. They would say things like, "I don't want you to help, I want Mom to help," because my wife would spend time with them while she got them ready for bed. Looking at the big picture, I realized that it took her longer, but the kids were happy.

Once I stopped assuming her intent, and thought about the big picture, I decided to talk with my wife instead of at her. I listened to her opinions and needs, and we came up with a solution. We decided that, if possible, we would get the children ready for bed together, and I would work afterwards. This way, we could get them into bed quickly AND happily. Also, I could think more clearly while working because I didn't have the background noise of tired children, or the stress of wondering why my wife hadn't put them to bed yet.

Here's another example. A client, Christy, found herself in a situation where she assumed her husband's intent. He would often visit the neighbor's house in the afternoon. He liked to socialize and talk, but would lose track of time. Often he would stay there for many hours, and she would have to call him home for dinner. Christy felt betrayed. As she saw it, her husband put socializing with the neighbors above spending time with the family. She felt he didn't care about her, because if did care, he would help get dinner ready, or at least play with his own children instead of the neighbor's. She assumed that he deliberately stayed for long periods of time. If he didn't come home, it was because he didn't care.

You can imagine the atmosphere in the house when her husband got home. Christy was reactive. When either party operates from a reactive place, misunderstandings and arguments follow. In order to resolve the situation, she needed to calm down, and ask her husband directly but politely to come home after a certain time. She also needed to remember that he wasn't deliberately trying to hurt her.

As I mentioned earlier, making assumptions is a reaction to stress. It happens when we don't think clearly about the situation. We need to remember that it is highly likely our partner's intentions differ from what we think. Sometimes, they are polar opposites. We can ask ourselves:

- "What's really bothering me in this situation?"
- "Is that worth having an argument about?"
- "What would be a better way to deal with this?"

In many cases, the better way to deal with a situation is to directly but politely ask for what you want. That leaves no room for interpretation–or misinterpretation.

The Infidelity Epidemic

Infidelity, or "cheating", continues to sweep the globe. There are many reasons why it happens: personal trials, one or both people waning in their commitment, the feeling of being ignored or underappreciated, or even bad decisions due to drunkenness. Some might follow in the footsteps of a childhood role model (such as a father, mother, or much older sibling). Others think it doesn't matter; after all, "everyone does this." Many blame their spouses or partners, pointing the finger at them because they don't want to do anything in the bedroom but sleep.

All of these scenarios reveal underlying factors. One that plays a big part, and generates plenty of stress from within the relationship, is comparing. It usually occurs when the two people face a challenge in their relationship. It could be a major situation, one that threatens to uproot the entire relationship, or the ups and downs of the day-to-day rhythm phase, when the excitement of the honeymoon period has passed and daily life feels ordinary, even mundane, lacking spark.

Let's say you or your partner meets someone – as a friend – and enjoys their company. The conversation is relaxed and fun, the laughter plentiful, and the constantly smiling face on the other side fresh and appealing. You make each other feel good. As you get to know this new person more, you might start comparing the good points of the friendship to the bad points of your relationship. What will shine more lustrously?

One of my clients, Sonja, was going through this process. Her husband, Victor, spent more and more time away from home after work. After working late at the office, he frequented a club or bar afterwards. When he arrived home, Sonja would ask, "Why were you out so long? Where were you?" Tension and conflict grew between them. There were other issues as well, common problems that couples experience and move through. Over time, communication, understanding of one another's feelings, and the "love" at home decreased. Sonja felt hurt and unimportant because of Victor's staying out so much. He felt guilty and untrusted because Sonja would question him.

Then Victor met Katrina. At first, they were just friends. But as the challenges at home increased, Victor spent more and more time at the club. His friendship with Katrina became more enjoyable. He started to compare the fun of their friendship with the challenges and lack of trust he faced at home. He felt that Katrina understood him, empathized with him. She consoled him about his troubles at home.

Meanwhile, his relationship with Sonja continued to deteriorate. She felt more and more hurt and became less and less trusting of him. Rather than respond to her concerns by coming straight home from work, or discussing their differences, Victor spent more and more time away, at the club, and with Katrina.

You can see what's coming next. This is how an affair develops–which it did. He and Katrina launched into an affair. Often, affairs start out with no bad intentions. Most people don't say, "Who can I find to have an affair with today?" It often starts out as a simple friendship with a co-worker, acquaintance, friend, or someone you meet in the course of your day.

Regardless of why the affair is happening, it's important to see the full picture. That includes looking at the new person–which would be Katrina, in Victor's case. Before the affair materialized physically, Victor was in an emotional, honeymoon-type period with Katrina. He only saw her good points. At the same time, he only saw Sonja's bad points. They were in the Day to Day phase of their relationship, and the rhythm was bumpy.

When Victor wouldn't stop having the affair, Sonja left him. She had loved him, taken care of him and met their challenges head on. She was a great woman. He lost her. He didn't care at the time, though: he had Katrina. After all, in his eyes, she stood for and provided everything Sonja did not.

However, when Victor and Katrina moved in together, a rude awakening soon awaited. Katrina pushed his buttons, too! And he pushed hers. Their balloon popped. Challenges arose. Victor was kicked back to square one. Again, he found himself in a relationship that needed work and maintenance (don't they all?). Again, he didn't take any actions or make himself available to keep the relationship strong. Katrina wasn't anywhere near as patient with him as Sonja. She left him in less than a year.

This process is why a very high percentage of relationships that begin with infidelity do not survive. When the truth comes out and both people see the full picture, they don't like what they see. Most cannot live with it. One or the other leaves. In addition, neither person has formed the skills necessary to keep a relationship alive. They soon do all the same things to their new partner that they did to their first, and the same challenges arise again. Infidelity, even if it seems fun at first, is never the answer.

Whenever you hold someone in higher esteem than your spouse or partner, recognize their weaknesses, too. If you were living with them, they would bother you just like your partner does–no matter how great you think they are. If you were to have an affair with them, you would most likely end up in the same place as the low point in your relationship that made you susceptible. Or lower.

To arrive at the full picture, look for the pros and cons of the situation. In addition, seriously reduce the amount of time you spend with the other person. If possible, stop spending time with them altogether. Best of all, if you really care about your partner and the longevity of your relationship, create a moral compass for yourself. Set a personal boundary that you will, *under no circumstances*, start an affair. Reinforce it as often as necessary. That way, when opportunities arise, you will have a pre-set boundary in place, never to be crossed. This simple act of advanced decision making has saved many, many relationships.

Here are some warning signs to let you know if you are on the path to having an affair. If you find yourself in any of these situations, it is time to take the steps described above:

- If you find yourself sharing feelings and thoughts with someone that you would normally share only with your partner
- If you find yourself feeling more appreciated, admired, or wanted by someone other than your partner
- If you appreciate, admire, or want someone else more than you want your partner

View your relationship from a different perspective. In particular, see the challenging times as an *opportunity* to learn how to keep your relationship strong. Work hard to make your relationship enjoyable again. Take more outings together. Spend more time in romantic settings. See your partner in ways you may not have seen him or her in years; create new freshness.

Search for the good in your partner. If you seek, you will find. It is much better to form the skills to keep a relationship strong, and to strengthen the relationship you have now, then to pass aimlessly from one fling to another. Far more often than not, affairs lead to despair and loneliness, associated stress and health problems–and unbearable regret.

Choosing to Grow and Forgive

Throughout the course of a relationship, it is practically impossible to be free of moments of hurt feelings, distrust, anger, and resentment. All of these will show up at different times–even when everything is going well. We've spent this chapter breaking down the many ways stress builds its destructive force from within the relationship and the ways we treat each other. Let's end on a strong note–the light at the end of the tunnel.

Every time relationship stressors occur, we have a choice. We can allow them to run (and potentially ruin) our lives, and be angry and resentful. Or, we can choose to resolve the problem and grow. Many stressful experiences are lessons in disguise. The same holds true within relationships. When our partner hurts our feelings, it is a good indication that something is amiss. It is an opportunity for us to grow personally and/or as a couple. We can choose to forgive.

As you read these words, you may be thinking, "How can I forgive him or her for hurting me like that? Insulting me? Taking it out on me? Messing with my life? You have no idea what they have done to me. I will never let this happen again." To which I say: don't worry. I'm not asking you to let them hurt you. Forgiveness isn't a green light for people to mistreat you over and over, then get away with it by saying, "I'm sorry," but rather, a process of releasing the hurt and resentment impacting *your* life. Forgiveness makes it possible for you to grow from the experience.

If left unchecked, resentment and anger burden and hurt us. When you hold onto anger and resentment and don't forgive, you give these negative emotions free rent inside your head, 24 hours a day, seven days a week. When you harbor hurt, and continue to let it fester, it impacts relationships and friendships negatively. Little problems look like you have focused a microscope on them. If you end up breaking up with the person who hurt you, and don't seek to understand the situation or forgive the person, it can (and probably will) impact any future relationship.

The first step to forgiving is to realize that the other person is a human being with baggage, too. They have their imbalanced perceptions. They learned things as children that aren't helpful to them now. They have suffered their fair share of pain and could be taking it out on you. Can you really expect them to be perfect? This in no way justifies their actions. It doesn't make wrong things right, but it does help you see things from their side. It also helps you to lend them the same degree of tolerance you would want for yourself. After all, you make mistakes, too.

The second step is to remember that good intentions aren't always followed by right actions. Sometimes, people do stupid things despite excellent intentions. Remember the maxim: "The road to hell is paved with good intentions?" In this situation, their actions could be a by-product of their own ignorance.

As stated earlier, this *does not mean* that you must let problems continue. For example, I would never recommend someone stay with an abusive partner, even if that partner offers up the best intentions–"I love you so much," "I won't do it again," "I can't believe I did that to you," etc. If they abuse once, they're likely to abuse again. If someone bothers or annoys you on a smaller scale, it is still best to learn and deal with the situation. When you realize that their intentions are likely not as bad as you think, it will help you resolve some of the resentment you feel towards them.

The third step is to recognize your own role in the situation. While it might seem the fault lies with your partner, there are possibly things that have done to contribute to the situation. Maybe you didn't set boundaries. Or, you took out subconscious or past pain on them. Perhaps you failed to communicate properly, or made a gruff comment under a moment of stress. The list goes on. All this causes stress for the other party, which might add to the stress they have caused you.

The fourth step is to learn and grow from the experience. Stressful experiences are an opportunity to learn. What is it you need to learn? To communicate your desires earlier on? Or in a more appropriate way? To stop putting unreasonable expectations on your partner? Or stop trying to live up to their unreasonable expectations? What is it?

Everything happens for a reason. Life is all about growth and education. What can you learn to help you become a stronger person? What can you learn to help your relationship become healthier?

When I was studying and working part time, one of my colleagues always complained about his wife. He complained about the way she treated him, and told me the different things she would do to hurt, upset, annoy or antagonize him. He started talking about leaving her, because he felt belittled with everything that she said. He jokingly talked about suing her for false advertising. After all, he told me, before they got married, they would go to the bedroom every time they saw each other. But once they got married, it was a rare occasion.

"Does that mean that she can sue you for false advertising?" I asked.

"It's not false advertising. I'm interested all the time," he said.

"Yes, but didn't you treat her with kindness, respect and love?"

"Yes," he said.

Then I asked if he still treated her the same way. For his response, he rattled off many excuses for treating her differently. I questioned him a little more, trying to help him see her side of the story better. As we discussed the problem, we found that his wife was doing similar things that his parents had done to him – actions which he had not yet learned to deal with yet. She pushed those same buttons. I taught him how to learn the lesson behind each button, and how to forgive. Now he had the chance to stop blaming and learn from it. His relationship with his parents and wife improved greatly.

The fifth step is to see the hidden benefit in the action your partner takes. Virtually every situation in life carries an obvious or hidden positive. Sometimes, our greatest victories come from our greatest challenges.

Remember the story of Rebecca in Chapter 2? Let's flash forward to the present. The change she has undergone is powerful. Her anger and lack of self worth from all the abuse in her life, and her inability to find someone to talk to, was so profound that her emotional body could no longer contain it; it manifested as a major thyroid growth that concerned her and doctors alike. It literally took away her ability to voice her concerns and to breathe. The physical manifestations of a childhood spent under the stifling oppression of the men in her life, and unable to cry out because her mother would punish her for crying. Once she identified the positives in her situation, her anger and fear of voicing her feelings or holding self-confidence subsided–and so did the tumor. It no longer had toxic emotions to feed it. By using these exercises and others including those in Chapter 8, she was able to gradually forgive the men who molested her.

Here are some of the exercises I gave Rebecca to help her confront her past and learn to move forward in her life:

1. Break Down Every Situation into Individual Elements

The first step is to break down the person who has upset you, or the situation itself, into different elements. For example,

Rebecca didn't like not being listened to by her mother, being violated, feeling dirty, the physical trauma, and the fact she had no choice. This will help with brainstorming the next step.

2. **Look for Benefits of the Situation**

Did you become independent? Do you now have a thirst for the good things in life which is opposite to what you experienced? What did you learn from it? How has it helped you? Are you a better friend, parent, partner or sibling because of the event? Are you more understanding? Once you have thought of 50 things about the event in general, visit those specific aspects of it that you thought of above. Now think of the benefits of each.

If this seems difficult, don't worry. For however long, your mind has only recognized the bad from a situation. Now you are forcing yourself to see the good part, something you have not been aware of yet. It is a completely different mental process. Carry on, because in the end, you will let go of hurt from the event. You will be able to move on. You will be able to live without that inner frustration, and be more capable of making clear decisions.

3. **Look Into Your Seven Aspects of Life: Physical, Financial, Family, Social, Vocational, Spiritual and Recreational**

When you feel you have come up with all possible benefits, take it further by looking into all areas of your life. Most likely, you have only seen how it has helped you in one to three areas. Look for benefits in the other areas as well.

4. **See the Benefits Within Those Benefits**

Start looking for the benefits of *those* benefits. For example, Rebecca found herself to be understanding and supportive of her children when events, similar to her own story, happened to them. It strengthened her relationship with her children. They did not need to endure as much pain as she did, and could begin their healing process more easily.

5. **Don't Stop Digging Until You See How Each Situation Was Equal Parts Problem and Blessing**

Keep going until you can see how the situation was equally a problem and a blessing. This does not make what happened right. It doesn't make it ideal. However, now you can see how you have received equal strength from the event, even though it hurt you greatly. You can let go of stress and resentment and enjoy the positives that have come out of the experience.

Chapter 5: Deep, Lasting Love: The Fortified Relationship

From time to time, we see couples remain as enthralled with each other as they were during their honeymoon period, more than a few Prime Ministers ago. They walk side-by-side, so happy to be with the person next to them, finding it impossible to imagine life without their partner. They laugh, converse easily and openly, find points in common no matter how far apart they are initially, and celebrate their togetherness.

Each of us knows a couple like this. Perhaps more than one. That couple might serve as a family bedrock, or the answer to one of life's most vexing questions: "How do they stay so happy after (you pick the number) of years?" The answer lies in the next question: "How have they been able to elevate their relationship above the stresses and challenges they've undoubtedly experienced?" Because they have. They have lived, worked and interacted with others in a society that is never at a loss for presenting stress-inducing situations. They have faced stresses within the home as well, from their spouse, kids, grandkids, or friends down the street. Some stresses could be flicked away as easily as a housefly. Others carried enough dynamite to potentially level a relationship if ignited.

Yet, they persevered. They rose above each and every stress. They came out of situations *stronger*, rather than damaged. They brushed off and moved forward *more* determined to hold their happiness together, rather than pointing fingers and talking about separation or divorce. In short, they acted as if their love and their relationship never touched the turbulent waters of a stressful world. It is a major reason why couples celebrate 25th, 35th, 40th, 50th and even up to 75th wedding anniversaries.

They're not only survivors, but also *thrivers*. They thrive on the lasting happiness, comfort and strength that awaits everyone who gets beyond the day-to-day effects of stress.

Like everything else, it takes plenty of trust and hard work. *By both parties.* As I've made clear in the past two chapters, the association between stress and any relationship not only exists, but can be quite devastating if you feed into it rather than working beyond it. Yet, when we figure out that each stressful situation gives us an opportunity to strengthen, rather than weaken, our relationships and ourselves, we can reach that hallowed place all couples seek as they grow older. It begins with setting the right behaviors and attitudes toward each other, the relationship, and each stressful situation as it unfolds.

Behaviors and Attitudes

When you enter a relationship, you bring along the attitudes, habits and behaviors formed over the previous years. You learned some of these from your parents. You picked up others from relatives, friends, the parents of your friends. Still others came from co-workers, musicians you listened to and watched in concert, and even people you watched on TV and movies.

At the same time, your partner arrives with their attitudes, habits and behaviors. No matter how young or old you are when the relationship begins, you come together like two huge circles of experiences. The key is to find out which behaviors and attitudes mesh. A lot of stress can occur from these learned behaviors if they are not helpful to relationships. For example:

- If you have learned to spend everything you earn and not budget your money, your relationship could suffer a lot of stress from financial challenges
- If you have not learned to control your temper, you could hurt your partner by saying or doing unkind things when the going gets tough

- If you have always received everything you want straight away, you may give up quickly when things become difficult or challenging. You may also have a hard time compromising with your partner, or accepting their opinion if it differs from yours
- If you have learned to always sacrifice your own needs for others, you may never get what you want in the relationship. You may eventually feel resentful and overpowered, and your partner may learn to take you for granted

Even though neither partner is deliberately trying to hurt the other, these problems can and do arise. It happens in every relationship, even those that exemplify "how to do it right". When you face challenges, it helps greatly to view them from a cause and effect perspective. Ask yourself:

- Is there any action, habit or way I'm living on my part that is causing this problem?
- What do I need to learn from this problem?
- How can I prevent it from happening again?

Be open and honest with yourself. After all, you are a good person. Most likely, you operate with the best intentions. However, you can't blame all of your relationship issues on your partner. In many cases, there are behaviors and attitudes on both sides that contribute to the problem. If you identify your part in the disagreement or conflict, you can change it and help the situation improve.

At the same time, *do not take responsibility* for your partner's role. There are two sides to every story, so the saying goes–and you can only adjust and correct your side. It is for the other person to see how their behavior or attitude is affecting your relationship. You can't blame all of your relationship issues on yourself. When you identify your partner's role, I guide against going on an active quest to change your partner. If necessary, work to set boundaries in a calm, kind way. For example, if your partner continues to dump every work problem on you (as if you can do anything about it, anyway!) and you resent and grow agitated from this nightly unloading, ask if he can keep the "debriefing" to five or ten minutes. That's usually enough time to release the steam and emotional toxins, and start to enjoy your time together. Once that time frame is agreed upon, you have a boundary.

Ask for what you want or what you think would help in the situation. Be open and direct about the problem and what you believe will solve it. Remind your partner that you are not blaming them. You could even ask them what they think will help solve the problem. Then adopt the behaviors and attitudes to move forward accordingly.

Remember: the arithmetic of relationships is not 1 vs. 1. It is not you versus your partner. It may feel that way, but in reality, it is 1 + 1, you *plus* your partner, ready to take on any problem together.

Setting Boundaries and Being Equally Yoked

Traditionally, women have had a problem setting boundaries. Much of this is due to many generations of social conditioning, in which the woman is taught to be submissive, and abdicate all authority to the "head of household". Without getting into particulars – and creating stress inside a book about *getting beyond* stress – the dynamics are a little different in the 21st century. Because of that, in today's society, both women and men need to set boundaries.

Back before cars, trucks and tractors, people used horses, carts, and wagons to get themselves to and from places. Horses pulled the wagons along most of the time. However, when you needed to move a big heavy load, you used oxen. The oxen would pull the load in pairs. When you hook up a pair of oxen to a cart, a heavy wooden bar would be placed over the top of their necks and fastened with wooden 'bows' around their throats. This is a yoke, and is what the load is attached to. It helps keep the oxen moving at the same pace and time, assuring a smoother rhythm. If one of the oxen is more powerful or stronger than the other, they are not equally yoked. One will pull harder, and the drivers will need to exercise considerably more effort to keep the wagon straight. If they do not, the unequally-yoked oxen may pull the wagon in a big circle.

The same thing can happen in a relationship. If one person does all of the work and the other doesn't "pull their weight", the relationship spins in circles. The solution for this is to give lovingly, while setting appropriate boundaries to ensure you don't give beyond your capacity.

A client story illustrates this point. Sarah came to my office to learn more about setting boundaries in her life. Some of her siblings were very unkind to her. They used and abused her by getting her to do excessive amounts of free work for them. This included babysitting their kids, running errands, picking things up for them, and a whole list of other time-consuming tasks and chores. She also followed their advice in making her life decisions, even though their advice stopped her from progressing. Their intentions were to keep her busy as their private servant! Sarah had a certain perception of her family: it was so important to her, that she was willing to give up her own life to help them be happy, even if it made her miserable. She was giving up her dreams, listening to what they said, and accepting their every word or opinion, even when not constructive for her.

Sarah reached the point where she was angry at her siblings and resented them for the way they treated her. She also was angry at herself for letting them treat her that way. Eventually, she moved to a different city to escape their influence. When the demands and requests crept back in, she moved interstate. She wouldn't call or visit, except on special occasions. This way, they could not use or influence her life anymore. However, the stress didn't completely leave–she was afraid of making life decisions that her siblings would disagree with.

I helped her to change her perspective on family. I helped her to see that family is important, but she needed to take care of herself first. She needed to learn to stand on her own two feet and to set boundaries. That started with a single word that so many of us find difficult to say, regardless of the situation or demand: NO. After she worked with that, she learned to do the things that were important for her, even if some of her family members didn't agree. Many of them felt uncomfortable when she finally said "no" to them. She stood up for herself and set her own goals.

You can guess what happened. Some of her family members became very resentful. They were very happy with the old Sarah, whom they could boss around and persuade to do their bidding. They lived at her expense, because she would reluctantly give up her plans to babysit their kids–so they could go out or fulfill their other plans instead. Suddenly, they felt some of the stress of responsibility that they had placed on her.

Not Sarah. She loved her new life. She felt free, important again, and able to finally achieve her goals. She is well on her way. Over time, her family members learned to accept that they couldn't treat her like a doormat anymore. Eventually, they learned to stop asking if they knew it would impose on Sarah's new outlook and attitude. More importantly, Sarah was also able to let go of her resentment towards her siblings, which made her feel a lot happier.

When we don't set boundaries or honor those of others, usually it amounts to one of two reasons. The first is a feeling of low self worth, as with Sarah. When a man or woman feels that he or she is not good enough, that person will give without asking for what they want or looking after themselves. If you want a healthy relationship that does not create undue stress, you must take care of your own needs and not allow your partner to overpower you. When you have feelings of low self worth, you are willing to let people treat you that way. In the long term, it creates resentment, feelings of not being appreciated and loved, and much less self-happiness. This creates stress, rather than reducing or eliminating it. But *you* hold the key: people can only impose their wills or wishes on you if you let them.

Sarah and I did a lot a lot of work on improving her self worth. Once she really knew what a great person she was, she found it almost easy to say "No". It still took courage on her part, but now she felt the courage, she saw the negatives to saying "Yes" in some of these situations–and she handled it well. I have outlined the rest of my work with Sarah in Chapter 8 on Self-Love. Aside from our one-on-one consultations, which I keep confidential, the exact program is there.

At this point, I want to emphasize the most important aspect of boundaries, so that you don't go crazy suddenly setting so many boundaries that they fence you in completely. That point is not directly about setting boundaries; it's about asking for support. Often, situations in which you feel taken for granted are resolved by asking for support. Always start off with this proactive mindset.

However, there are situations where asking for support isn't enough. In these situations you need to set boundaries. The giving and receiving of assistance is a boundary. It's not talked about as often as communication or self-worth boundaries, but it needs to be understood and established nonetheless if you want a relationship beyond stress. Men will do best to remember that women love to receive offers of help. Just a few times can make a difference. Women, you need to remember that men trust you. When you need help, ask. Be polite, kind, and direct. Men often don't want or need explanations. In fact, explanations can come across to the male ego and mind as blame. Ask, "Would you please do the dishes tonight?" as opposed to "I'm so tired. This house is always a mess. I do so much work around here! Would you please do the dishes tonight?"

Don't wait until you are desperate. Ask during a period when it will still be OK if they say "No". That way, you won't explode. You can ask again a little later (if you still need help), directly and politely saying something like, "Look, I really need a hand, when can you help me?" Above all, when they do help, show the necessary appreciation they deserve. Appreciation is king.

You can also politely say "No" when your partner asks too much of you. So long as you communicate with openness, saying no is not an insult.

When setting boundaries, it's important to remember that your partner still loves you. There is a large chance that they continually cross into your space with the best intentions. Don't view them as an enemy. Speak to them in the same way as you do when you are not frustrated or irritated.

Set boundaries politely, calmly and assertively. Do so in a spirit of mutual accomplishment; in other words, after you've laid down the boundary you want to set, ask your partner, "Is there something I'm doing to get into your space that you'd like me to know about?" Expecting more from your partner and giving less can create conflict itself. It's important to communicate this change without attacking.

Understanding Each Other's Priorities and Values

In relationships, there are many things to learn about our loved ones – and ourselves. If your eyes, mind and heart are open, you can probably find something new most every day. One very important thing to learn concerns your partner's priorities – and your own. If you don't know the priorities, beliefs and values your partner elevates above all else, you can easily become frustrated with their behaviors, and vice versa. It also causes misunderstandings, where gestures of love are ignored or even taken the wrong way. That leads to conflict. Learning each other's priorities will help you understand your partner's behavior better. With that it's easier to negotiate and form better situations when you both know what's important to each other.

A client of mine, Vanessa, was considering divorce. After almost 30 years of marriage, she felt her husband no longer loved or cared about her. He never gave her flowers, nor did he spend much time with her. When they were together, he would watch football on TV. She would leave the room or even the house, because she didn't care about football. The fire in their relationship was gone. She didn't feel appreciated or wanted.

I was also helping her with other stresses in her life. I asked her what her husband valued, what was important to him. "Sports and watching sports" she said, among other things. He even invited her to watch sports with him on TV, but she said no, because she thought he didn't care.

I pointed out to her that while he definitely wasn't thoughtful, he did love her. However, he wasn't showing the love through the things she valued and cared about. She valued flowers, special dates, and time together talking. But, he wasn't doing those things. He was only showing that he loved her in the things that mattered to him. He felt that asking her to join him for some football on the TV was both important and a gesture of love. He invited her out of respect and love. It also turned out he also valued money, to be more specific, not spending it. That is why he never bought her flowers.

By understanding what her husband valued, Vanessa came to see that he did still love her. She felt so much relief. She even started accepting his offers to watch football on TV with him. She didn't want to divorce him anymore.

In time, her husband reciprocated. Just by Vanessa showing him supportive love in the things he considered important, he became fonder of her. Beforehand, he didn't show much affection of any sort. She communicated this to him, but he would always dismiss it. Now, he puts his arm around her in a very affectionate way. Amazingly, he even does the dishes!

Vanessa was very impressed with that. He went out of his way to pick her up from the train station when it was raining, so that she didn't have to catch a bus home (before, she caught a bus, even if he was at home). They still have other challenges, but they overcame a big hurdle.

Vanessa's example shows the long term damage that can come from not knowing each other's priorities. It seems extreme, in that she was willing to divorce her husband over a small problem and thoughtlessness that had grown over many years. But even in smaller cases, knowing each other's priorities and values can still have big effects. This knowledge can help build the fire of a relationship over the long run, add understanding, and create more effective communication. On the flip side, the misunderstandings caused by not knowing each other's priorities can only slowly douse the flames of love, create resentment, hurt and anger.

Let's look at the traditional stereotypical relationship with the working dad and stay-at-home mom. The woman may complain that the man works too many hours, and does not spend enough time at home with her and the kids. Many husbands will counter by saying that she doesn't respect him, nor does she realize how important it is for him to work so hard, so constantly, to pay the bills, pay for sports activities and feed college funds.

The woman values kids and family highly. The man values career and finances. Once they get past their complaints, and start to see it from the others' perspective and that of the relationship and family, their stress reduces. Why? Because they realize how they help each other. The man earns money that pays for food, clothing, bills and activities for the children. The woman puts a lot of effort and time into raising the children. Her efforts mean that he can relax more when he gets home. His efforts mean that she can breathe more easily, knowing that she won't be looking for food or a place to live, and that she will be covered when she grows older.

When we recognize how our priorities help each other, we appreciate each other more, become more forgiving, and less likely to resort to conflict. We can still ask for more time with the kids, or a break from the kids, but it is a good starting point.

How to Learn Yours and Your Partner's Priorities and Values

A quick way to learn and understand our priorities is by looking at what we like and dislike, the most and least important things, and the actions we take and don't take.

To find out what you prioritize, ask yourself the following questions. Write down the first three answers that come to you:

- o What do you spend your time doing?
- o What are you willing to spend money on?
- o What do you think about in your spare time?
- o What do you like talking about (with each other, with friends)?
- o What do you like reading about?
- o What are your favorite magazines?
- o What are your favorite forms of music? Or bands?
- o What are you disciplined and most competent in?
- o What are your goals?

Collect your answers and sort them into categories: financial, career, recreational, relationships and family, spiritual, mental or educational, physical or health. The categories that contain the most answers are those most important to you. This shows what we really value.

There is often a difference between what we want to prioritize, think we prioritize, and *actually prioritize*. You might think you value your partner, but your actions might not show it. The example of Vanessa and her husband illustrates that. Knowing your priorities and those of your partner allows you to adjust your actions to honor the things important to them.

When you understand your partner's values, you will better see how your partner is showing love to you. You will also recognize how they support the things you prioritize. You will appreciate and admire them more, which in itself will resolve some of the hurt and resentment. This reduces the debilitating stress that boils from within a relationship.

Conflict is a Reaction

Any form of conflict causes stress. When that conflict grows and festers, the stress builds. Your life outside the home could be the smoothest, most enjoyable and stress-free you have known, but if you and your partner are constantly in conflict, it will likely dampen everything else. When conflict happens between partners, it can be emotionally and mentally paralyzing.

Conflict begins with a *reaction*. When you feel angry and continue to argue, even to the point of liking it, you are usually seeing only one side of the story. You are reacting to the side you see. Your feelings are not based on the full picture. If they were, chances are you wouldn't be so upset.

At the same time, other factors influence your feelings. Your stress levels could already be high. Maybe you are tired, under pressure at work, or "having a bad day". The situation causing the conflict at home could remind you of a past hurt. Or, it could tap into a deep, hidden fear.

When your anger or frustration rises, and you sense an argument brewing, ask yourself:

- "Why am I really upset?"
- "How did I feel before this argument? Was I already upset about something else?"
- "Is there anything else going on at the moment that is stressful to me?"
- "Could that be influencing the way I feel now?"

Asking and answering these questions will help you to rein in your emotions. You may feel a lot less frustrated with the current issue, because the insights you gain will help you see things more clearly. Even if you still feel stressed, you will have more awareness and control over your response to the situation. Your partner could be experiencing the same feelings of frustration, anger and tunnel vision, too. Perhaps they have had a bad day, feel plenty of pressure from work, or have some other situation stressing them out. When you realize that the same process could be happening with them, try not to take their reactions personally. While their anger may be taken out on you, in many cases, the real source of their stress has nothing to do with you. They were likely within one degree of the boiling point already, and your small action tipped them over. In psychology, this is known as displacement[3].

Negotiating and Compromise

One of the most vital conflict resolution skills for any relationship is the ability to negotiate and compromise. It is natural that you will disagree from time to time. When this happens, you can:

    a. Push what you want on your partner; or

    b. Learn what they want, and compromise

While pushing and imposing your will allow you to prevail in the short term, in the long haul it will create feelings of being controlled and oppressed. That results in conflict. While compromising may be tough at first, its benefits are worth it.

When I was growing up, my dad always said to me: "Do you want to be right, or do you want to be married?" What he meant was this: when you have an argument, and try your hardest to make your partner see that you are right and they are wrong, you threaten your relationship. You could both even be hurtful and say things you will regret later.

In an argument, no matter how right you both think you are–and in point of fact, one or both of you may be *factually correct*–both are inevitably *wrong*. Why? Because you leave no room for an answer to suit both of you. You won't listen to each other. While your point might seem right, your way of delivering it is wrong. You are both trying to win the argument, but in so doing, losing each other's respect and trust, and igniting high levels of stress. What matters most?

Disagreements are an unavoidable part of any relationship– an opportunity to learn more about each other and to grow stronger. However, uncompromising conflict is no way to deal with it. The anger response only creates hurt, both in the short and long run. By listening and compromising, you can resolve a lot of conflict–an idea which I explore more deeply in the next section.

Let's look at a potentially worst case scenario: what do you do when listening and compromising aren't enough? I once saw an elderly couple on TV. They had just celebrated their 50th wedding anniversary. The reporter asked them what their secret was to a long and happy relationship. The husband's answer? "Yes, dear."

Men have a good laugh over this response. However, in this case, the husband long ago felt it was better to quickly fizzle out an argument than let it continue and build up. He was willing to say yes to anything his wife asked. I think this response is perfectly appropriate when a woman is venting. "Yes, dear" proves to her that you are not only listening, but that you care.

Sometimes, though, saying "Yes, dear" isn't enough. Especially when you want something specific for your own happiness or peace of mind. In these situations, it is still better to end the conflict quickly. If listening isn't working, or you find yourself unable to listen without getting worked up, you can end the conflict with: "I can see this is just going to hurt both of us.

It isn't going anywhere good. I'm going to take a walk, and once we've calmed down, we can discuss it properly."

Taking a walk or moving to another room physically removes you from the argument. It reduces stress and tension, which opens up the channels for communication, listening, and compromise. While your partner might not like it at first, as they calm down, they will see the reason why you took this action and appreciate you more for it. It gives you time to calm down and properly think about things. You can reassure your partner at the same time with a statement like: "I love you. I can see that we're both going to get hurt from this. I don't want to hurt you, so I'm going to go for a walk to calm down. Later on, we can discuss it peacefully."

Finally, learn how *not* to argue. My wife and I do not often argue, but when we do, we both are capable of running our disagreement into a hurtful place neither of us wants to visit. However, it almost never happens. Speaking for myself, when an argument between us continues for even a minute or two, I choose to remain silent until I have calmed down. Another approach might be to stop, pull back and ask yourself, "What is trying to happen here?" Gain some immediate perspective. Don't fall into the flash fire of the moment. If you can take a step back, and not make that next point, then you will stop the vast majority of arguments in their tracks. Another conflict resolved!

Effective Listening Is Critical to the Art of Compromise

"You have two ears and one mouth; use them in that order."

Listening is vital to communication. That's the second half of the equation, right? One person talks, the other listens. Quite often, it's more important than speaking. Listening becomes even more essential when two people disagree. When you listen, you can find out what your partner really wants. When you know what your partner really wants, you are better equipped to arrive at a solution that fills both of your needs.

There is more. Much more. When you listen to your partner, something amazing often happens: their resistance to whatever is bugging them lowers. They no longer feel the need to push their opinion across so strongly, because you are listening. They can communicate their wants more constructively. That opens the door for you to communicate your wants, and to have a conversation, which results in compromise: both people receiving beneficially because the other is willing to give.

For example, the following situation is a common experience for men. You might want to go out with friends tonight, but your partner wants you to stay home with the family. The conversation might proceed like this: "I want you to stay home with us. You never stay home with us. You always go out with your friends."

Not a lot of room for response, is there? You may not even have to ask why. Women will naturally say WHY they think a certain way; in an argument, the trick is to listen and not take blame. This makes it easy to see that your partner's real desire is for you to spend more time together. Maybe time with family is high on their priorities list, and you are not fulfilling it. Because of this, they may feel unimportant.

If you listen to the meaning behind their words, and know their priorities, you can give back from within those priorities. That will make your partner more trusting and willing to honor items that are high on your list of priorities. With reassurance, and compromise, they may relent so you can go out–for the one night. Don't presume that it means all other nights, too. It doesn't. Do something special with the family the next night, or vice versa. Reassure your partner of their importance to you by giving them something that feeds their values and priorities. By compromising through active, effective listening, you validate each other's needs.

The next step is to communicate in a way that shows your partner how the solution will benefit them. To make this even more effective, talk in terms of your partner's priorities. In the above situation, you could say, "I can see how you want me to stay home more. How about we do something special tomorrow and the next evening? You can choose, or I'll come up with some surprises."

If she says, "Well, I don't know … neither one of us has had any good ideas lately," or something like that, be ready with a positive response that serves both of you. An example: "I still want to go out with my friends tonight. While I'm out, I'll ask them what surprises they've done for their family. But in the end, you will still get to decide."

If you put it to your partner like that, even *they* will find your night with friends appealing.

Let me share another example. Let's say a guy wants to buy a new car that he has long wanted and coveted. I'm sure the vast majority of marriages and relationships know this one! The man could say, "I'm getting the car because I like it."

Whether she dislikes the color, style, lack of space for the kids, or the sticker price, won't really matter. If you declare your intention to buy the car with these words, you will get some blowback. If your partner does not value cars at all, but does treasure time with you, the purchase will not appeal to her. She may fear that joyrides into the country will steal away your precious time together. She knows that once you get into that car, she will struggle to get you out of it.

It all adds up. "No," she says, her uncompromising tone just as strong as your uncompromising statement that you're going to buy the car. She will resist because it threatens her higher priority–time with you. Along with that, she will likely point out her other concerns.

On the other hand, if you know and understand that her priorities do not include cars that suit your fancy, you might say,

"I'm looking at getting this new sports car. It's a two-seater, and it will be our hot date car. We can go out and spend some time with each other, we can go out to dinner and talk, and just enjoy each other's company." Suddenly, your description appeals to her. You've also listened to her and know her priorities, because you captured her biggest need in your statement–spending more quality time together. She may suddenly see this new car idea as a good idea.

Since we're looking at how to find stress-free compromise, I will now turn the tables. Let's say you, as a woman, want to get a new necklace, with matching earrings. You know that your partner thinks you have enough jewelry, and he values money highly. However, you listen to your partner and know how to blend together your priorities and desires with his concerns – and the things that make him happy. You might say, "I am looking at getting this necklace. It is beautiful and I really like it. It will look really good for you at the next business dinner. It will show that you are doing well and could influence more people to do business with you."

What an appealing approach! It certainly sounds much better and more beneficial to both partners than, "I want to get a new necklace and I'm getting it", (or, "I want that car because I've always wanted to race around the outback"). He may initially value the necklace as an investment – his normal justification for buying such an expensive item. However, through your loving comments, he can see how it would make you sparkle, feel better about yourself. Which makes him feel better about himself – and the both of you. Here we have a win-win situation.

Use this communication technique to reach solutions that suit both of you. Keep your side of the commitment. Be honest with your partner and follow through on what you've said you will do. Mutual trust will reign the next time you compromise.

Remember: your needs and your partner's are equally important. Both sets of opinions are valid. Both ways of thinking add to the relationship. When you compromise, you make the relationship deeper. And, you increase your happiness–which reduces stress.

Giving Up Control

Controlling relationships occur when one person imposes their will on the other, repeatedly. No matter what the source of the controlling dynamic (I list a few below), nothing is more potentially damaging, destructive or abusive than control. When left unchecked, control not only is stressful, but potentially dangerous.

Sometimes, a controlling situation is set up because of communication problems, or a perceived difference in success or stature between partners. One partner might be embarrassed about the other, or doesn't want them to look bad in front of family or friends. So they may tell their partner what to do to avoid embarrassment.

Another reason that controlling others arises ... is from good intentions. Perhaps there is an issue, and they think they have a good solution. If their partner doesn't agree, they may resort to control techniques to try and get what they want. Or, one partner or the other is used to getting their way all the time. Perhaps they are mirroring the example of parents or others. They haven't learned to compromise, so they resort to control techniques. They haven't learned to be happy when they don't get what they want.

When someone or something pushes a partner's buttons or reveals a deep-seated fear, that person can employ control techniques to push away and avoid their real or perceived fear. Stress rears its ugly head in this scenario in a big way: an otherwise calm, fair and relaxed person can become an anally-retentive control freak when buttons are pushed and fears are kicked up.

This leads to the biggest reason why people control others: to compensate for a feeling of lack of control in their own lives. When someone controls and dominates, you can bet something inside themselves, or in their lives, is running amok.

Controlling breaks down relationships with explosions of resentment and hurt feelings. Even mild forms of control, such as bossing around, nagging, and slight manipulation, reduce closeness and intimacy. More extreme forms, such as aggression, physical domineering, and withholding of money, sex or other privileges, destroy trust. Destructive and/or dangerous situations can arise if you don't address them.

Giving

Do you remember when you first met your partner? Remember all of the thoughtful things you did for them, and they for you? Those special notions of appreciation, thanks and admiration? Maybe you walked to the passenger's side of the car and opened the door. Or made reservations at *the other person's* favorite restaurant? Maybe you put on music they liked. Or sat and listened to their opinions, their life experiences, for an entire evening. Gave them a foot or shoulder massage. Or filled them with compliments about how they looked, thought, spoke, or otherwise brightened up your life.

Remember how you and your partner's eyes would then meet, gazing into the other, feeling like time stood still? You didn't even have to say the three words, "I love you," because it was already etched into your expressions. What a gift–to you, to the other, to both of you.

Giving is an essential part of a healthy relationship. Taking time to deliberately give to your loved one keeps the passion alive and builds it for the long term. Your partner feels wanted, admired, appreciated, cherished and trusted. This creates more love and helps a relationship withstand rocky periods. When a problem arises, it is much easier to remedy if both parties feel loved, cared about and important.

Once you know what is important to your loved one, you can give freely and openly, in a more fulfilling way. Sometimes, though, people go into relationships with the wrong idea, i.e. "What's in it for me?" They view each other as the answer to their dreams, or fulfillment of their greatest financial or emotional desires–and will focus almost entirely on that prize. In the long run, this creates resentment. One party (or both) may have unreasonable expectations of the other. They get resentful when their expectations are not met. The other party feels taken for granted and becomes resentful, too. Either way, the floodgates of stress swing open and put a huge damper on the future.

Within relationships, there are two primary ways to give. The first involves those everyday things that need to be addressed when living together. This includes taking out the trash, cooking, mowing, working, raising children, etc.

The spirit of giving means reframing those day-to-day tasks, projects or actions that you take on. When you give, handle these tasks with the attitude of, "I'm doing this because I love you", instead of, "I'm doing this because I have to". Ever notice the difference those two statements make in the approach you take to cooking dinner or washing dishes? When you operate from a spirit of giving, you won't grow resentful of all those basic responsibilities that are part of a living together relationship–and sometimes, handling the other's tasks as well as your own.

Giving also involves putting in the effort that shows your partner you love them. These kind little gestures can include an extra smile, a hug and kiss when they get home, maybe reading poetry or a favored passage to them, drawing a special bath with oils and candles, things like that.

The reward of giving is to experience the other's happiness. You see the joyous smile on their face, and the appreciation in their eyes. It came from your action. You care about their happiness, and they know it. When they feel that appreciation, a chemical change happens within the brain[4]. It creates the desire for them to more completely fulfill your needs, wants and desires. The relationship continues to grow stronger. I also talked about this in Chapter 3.

When you know your loved one's priorities and values, you can give them something they value highly. That will endear you even more to them, and bring more depth and joy to your love. For example, if your loved one values family, you could make an extra effort to spend time doing something the whole family enjoys. If your partner values health and fitness, you could give them extra workout time, join them at the pool, or tell them how great they look when exercising. If your loved one values working, you could thank them for providing financially, and maybe pack a nice lunch for them. The possibilities are limited only by your imagination and what would be thoughtful and considerate for your partner.

These twelve acts of giving suit most partners very well, and serve as a nice go-to list if you do not have other ideas:

1. Flowers (for women)
2. Help with the housework
3. A massage, or a massage voucher
4. A night off with friends
5. A note of appreciation or admiration
6. A sincere compliment in the morning
7. Saying "I love you" and meaning it
8. Making their favorite dinner, lunch or breakfast to have together
9. Taking them on a surprise date to do something they enjoy

10. A note expressing thanks for the things they do

11. A gift they will enjoy

12. Doing one of their "chores" every now and then as a surprise

Love Yourself

To enjoy a really happy relationship, you must learn to love yourself. That is easier said than done, especially when some in our growing-up years, parents, ministers, teachers and schoolmates may have filled us with the opinion that "only selfish people love themselves."

The lack of self-love leads to a life path well worth leaving. When you lack self love, you often accept partners who mistreat you. At first, you won't be bothered by it, but as time goes on, you will resent them. If it happens with more than one relationship, you probably will think, "All men/women are the same", and wonder if there are any good potential partners out there. You might also ask, repeatedly, "Why do I keep ending up with people who mistreat me?" Why? Because deep down, you do not think you deserve better. On the outside, you will say, "Of course I deserve better." In your heart, however, you might have a hard time thinking of just ten good things to say about yourself. Do you constantly cut yourself down? Feel like you were meant to always hurt? Those thoughts indicate the opinion that you deserve less than the best.

Your relationship might be healthy now, but if you are not happy with own yourself, you and your partner will move into conflict more easily. When that happens, you probably won't look on the bright side of things. You may have a hard time standing up for yourself, or you may even overcompensate by controlling others.

When you love each other, and feed each other more *because* you also love yourself, happiness ascends to the front of your relationship and stress flinches and hides like a thief in the shadows. And that's what we all truly want in relationship: a union that stress cannot bend or break. I discuss this much more thoroughly in Chapter 8.

Chapter 6: The Workplace

You enjoy a fabulous weekend, filled with friends, a sports event, maybe a performing arts show or movie, and a party. Your kids even make you breakfast in bed. You and your spouse thoroughly enjoy each other's company, finding the weekend a perfect time to shrug off the stresses of the week and focus on what makes your relationship strong and enduring. As you drive into work Monday morning, relaxed and calm from your weekend, nothing can dampen your lofty spirit and feeling of goodwill and success.

Or can it? By noontime, you wonder why you ever left the house. The boss has already tossed three deadline projects on your desk that didn't exist Friday evening. Another client is blaming you for a sub-standard performance that did not involve you at all. Your to-do list looks more like a novel than a short series of tasks. Nonetheless, you seize the first sudden project with great initiative and scope, putting your skills to work – but are interrupted by phone calls and people popping their heads into your office.

By the time you get to the third project, your weekend glow is gone. You are uptight, barking at co-workers, wishing your boss had taken a one-way flight to Antarctica over the weekend (a perfect climatic match for his or her personality, you quip to yourself), and racing through your tasks with none of your earlier creative initiative. You rub your forehead–often–and feel every bone and muscle in your body constrict.

Then, just when you think you have survived this back-to-work day and can unwind the stress inside that has risen from non-existence to powder keg status in eight long hours, the boss walks through the door: "John, we need you to represent us at XYZ's company dinner tonight."

"Can my wife go?" you ask.

"No. This is strictly a business dinner."

Your irritation graduates to anger. You've put up with stressful weeks for so long and managed to relax on weekends because of a great home environment, but now it's back into the hornet's nest–where it never seems to stop. Unless you want to live in self-chosen poverty, or find a better financial or workplace alternative, this is likely a course on which you need to stay for the next ten, twenty or thirty years. Maybe more.

Welcome to the workplace. Along with financial pressures, it is the leading source and cause of stress. It also is probably the one stress-causing element of our lives over which we have the least control, unless we own or run the company or business. Others make decisions that create more responsibilities for us. We work to the deadlines and expectations of our superiors, clients, or the dictates of the projects themselves. Any mistake we make leads to a negative result – and greater stress. A bad mistake can cost us our job. To top it off, we need to perform with our co-workers, whether or not we personally like them.

A challenge? Absolutely. What really becomes challenging, though, is when that workplace stress comes home with you. If everything is good at home, and your relationship strong and happy, it can and will mitigate the workplace stress. However, if you have other issues, then workplace stress can become unhealthy, even crippling.

This chapter covers common stressors at the workplace–both practical and deeper issues and challenges. While we don't often have control over events at work that cause stress, we do have control over how we react and respond.

That's where looking at workplace stress through the prism of our own lives comes in. For instance, with the gossip and bullying sections I present later in the chapter, one thing to ask yourself is, "Where have I seen this before in my life?" It may be the merry-go-round effect, the same issue coming around again because you haven't learnt from it. You can use this self-examination when mulling over the points in this chapter.

Look for what you need to learn. This is important. Do you need to be more assertive? Do you need to focus better and ignore or brush off unwarranted criticism? Can you find more effective ways to resolve conflicts, and keep them resolved? Can you do a better job of clocking out at normal time so you can get home to your family and not be sucked into the "long-hour blues"?

One thing you probably have learned already about my approach to a less stressful life: everything that creates stress in our lives has deeper root causes. The workplace is no exception. Strike a balance between work and personal life.

Balancing Act

Some people use work as a way to escape from their stress. In an American television movie of the late 1990s, this point is made clear by a wife who chides her husband for not spending more time at home with herself and the kids: "I have to go to work now," he says. "You have to go to escape," she replies.

In modern society, a lot is expected of us professionally, but we need to create and maintain balance in our lives. Whether employed or self-employed, we need to understand that work is just a necessary part of life–not the full picture.

I have noticed that many people seem to have two marriages running at the same time–one to the person they love, the other to their job. Unfortunately, more than a few put greater effort and energy into growing the work "marriage" than the one that involves rings, a ceremony, and lifelong vows!

In my work, and from personal observation, I notice that many of those married to the job reach this concerning point due to some sort of stress in their life. Many times, the stress arises from a financial issue. People think they have to work hard to earn money. True, but working hard is different than working yourself into the ground. Sometimes, this need to work to the bone comes from the fear that if they do not put in long hours, they may not have a job or, they might go bankrupt. Sometimes, they use the job to disguise a relationship issue. Maybe another area in life leaves them feeling a lack. To hide from that stress, they bury their heads in work and rarely come up for air.

I consulted with a client who was married to his work. He often started around 5:30 a.m. and didn't finish until at least 5 p.m. He commonly worked as late as 7 p.m. A 12- to 14-hour day was normal to him, including the same hours on most Saturdays. He was one of those people to which admiring bosses point and say, "He's working 24/7."

After we started working together, I asked him some questions. Soon, he realized exactly when he started working like this–it was when his wife suddenly left him. She took their young daughter and son and ran off with another man. He did not get to see his children, whom he dearly loved, for another fourteen years. Therefore, he had nothing to do with their upbringing. By the time my client reacquainted with his daughter, she had become a drug addict with major issues. He was doing everything he could to help, because he wanted to build a proper relationship with her and help her to straighten out her life. She chose not to accept his help.

In working with me, my client started to see that he could reclaim his personal life and find other forms of fulfillment and satisfaction. He stopped working long hours, but it took a lot of self-discipline. He was deeply married to his job for many years. He had used all those hours to hide from the hurt he felt from his wife leaving him.

Work is a means to an end, but it's not the end. Life isn't just about working. We need to work to make it financially easier to achieve our goals, dreams and desires, but it doesn't mean we dream to work.

Others work long hours, but it's not their choice. Often, they want to spend more time at home with their families, or relax with friends. However, it seems there is no other way to pay the bills, grow the college funds, or take care of investments. The list goes on. If this is you, the next section will certainly help.

Clocking Off

When the workday ends, home time begins. Or, it ought to. It is time to leave the office and return home, not just physically, but mentally and emotionally as well. If we live alone, then we need to take care of ourselves, maybe make a nice little dinner, exercise for a while, visit with the neighbors, listen to some music or watch a good movie. If there are others at home, then we need to take care of them as well–*and allow them to care for us.*

I used to commute to the office by train. I used that travel time to go over my day, both stressful and enjoyable events, and what I needed to do to fix it the next day. After that, I used the rest of the hour-long train ride to relax. Later, when I was driving, instead of allowing myself to get angry at the crazy and senseless ways other people were zipping around on the roads, I used the time to wind down.

Clocking off means exactly that: when you finish work, begin to throttle down. Start while heading home. On your drive, if your commute to work is not long and you still need to wind down a little more, sit around the corner, or sit at a park to finish winding down. Find a spot to wind down, so that once you walk through your front door, you are present *at home.* You might even think of ten good things that happened during the day, and slip into the pleasant energy of those events when walking inside your home.

Winding down helps prevent you from dumping the stress of your day on family members. They already have their own stresses. It is unfair to expect your spouse and kids to drop their own causes, concerns or responsibilities, and come rushing to you because your day was stressful. If they *choose* to comfort you, that is another story. But it's their choice, not yours.

I knew of a man who mentally hung his stress on a large tree in his front yard just before walking in the door. On one occasion, when his business had been burglarized and a sum of money went missing, he followed his normal routine, laid both burglar and financial impact to rest in the upper branches, and walked in the door as though his day had been the same as any other. He became present with his family. The next morning, before heading to work, he returned to the tree to mentally take the stress back, and found it was not as bad as he had thought. He told me that he noticed how much the stress lightened between evening and the next morning.

This technique may work for you–or you may need something else. The point is, you need to find a way that works for you. Meditation may be the answer. Perhaps you can review what caused your stress, why it stressed you, and why you responded or reacted as you did. What can you do better the next time it happens? When that next time happens, and it will, deal with it in a better way. You can use the questioning techniques in Chapter 1. Start the evening with a clean slate, and work hard to not hold onto the stress you experienced at work.

Another tip: if you have a work number, turn off the phone when you get home. If it is a phone that you can't disconnect, make a commitment that you will not take any more business calls after you get home. Many of my clients and friends who ignore this step find themselves thinking "Wow, I'm having a good time, but my phone could ring any minute." If the phone does ring, they immediately focus on the call and stop being present in their current activity, or family time. If they answer, they are too busy thinking about what actions they will need to take. Once you get home, be fully present. Enjoy being home. After all, you have earned it.

Showing Up

This section concerns our ability to be mentally present and focused at work, to give our best. Being mentally present won't solve all your stresses. For instance, your boss or a client might make insatiable demands on you, no matter how great your products are or how exemplary the work on a report you turned in. However, you can leave work each day happy with yourself, knowing that you showed up and gave your best. You don't have to worry about your boss getting frustrated with you all the time. This also opens up opportunities for advancement.

If you are employed and collecting a paycheck, it is best to be steadfastly loyal to the company that employs you. This is not only appropriate, but also reduces your stress. Be grateful that someone has given you the opportunity to utilize your skills, while helping you pay your bills and look after yourself. This is an important work ethic. It helps you to focus and perform at your best. When you're focused, outside distractions slow to a minimum. Just as you need to be fully present when you get home, when you start work, you need to be fully present and focused.

Appreciate the opportunity you have been given. I do not mean to brown nose or throw yourself at your boss' feet and become a doormat. I am not saying to be a "Yes Sir, three bags full" employee, nor am I saying to let your employer mistreat or disrespect you. However, you owe it to the company to do your best and focus on the task in front of you. Give it 100 percent. Everything else in life can wait until you are finished, unless it is an emergency. Likewise, if you are self-employed, focus on the projects and tasks for which your customers and clients are paying you. Self-employed people tend to be more motivated than employees, for one reason–if they don't perform, they lose their clients. Employees often receive more cushion than that, but there is no excuse for poor, unfocused performance. It also creates undue stress.

Fulfill your work duties efficiently so that the company can serve customers with great service and run smoothly. This approach can open up opportunities to progress in your area, as well as pay rises and promotions. For most people, advancement brings along reduced stress.

When I was working with a stockbroking firm, I had just been given a promotion and was doing my job very efficiently. My team and team managers were really happy with me, but then they started to expect that sort of effort from me on a daily basis. During that time, a colleague and I worked closely together. We had to swap paperwork back and forth to get our jobs done. Problem was, he was often away sick, and I would need to handle his work if I wanted to finish my own. The team managers were supposed to pick up the slack, but they already had their own work and could only get to his duties sometimes. Because he was away so much, it came to a point that I could actually perform both of our jobs. However, it created more stress than I wanted.

That didn't matter to the company. They decided to fire him and put me in charge of both jobs. Great! Surely they would give me a good pay rise. We were being paid the same, so I looked forward to receiving the extra wage. That's not what happened. I was in a very good place with my team managers and we worked together well, but I didn't know the big boss. He only knew that I worked hard. He said that he wanted me to take on the second role–without a pay increase. I had been told he had a sense of humor, so at first I thought he was joking. When I realized that he wasn't, I told him I didn't want to do both jobs if I wasn't going to be compensated more. It meant I would have to work twice as hard with no extra reward. I would carry a lot of overtime without being paid for it, so I had many concerns with this idea. "Well, this is how we're doing it," he said.

I responded by saying that they either gave me a fair pay rise, or I would not assume the extra role. He told me that it was out of the question … that I was not going to be paid my former colleague's salary as well as my own. He continued to remind me that I was a lower employee and that I would be paid the lower rate. I decided to compromise. If he would meet me halfway, I said, then I would consider the opportunity. He disagreed, so I let him know that my contract did not include this extra workload, and he would have to hire someone else for that role. He continued trying to threaten and bully me, so I showed him a copy of my contract. When my immediate managers found out what happened between the big boss and me, they were shocked– but respected my way of handling it, and why I felt the way I did.

I was loyal to the company. I worked hard, doing more than my job required, and helping others finish their jobs more effectively. However, when the big boss tried to strong-arm me into doing more work without extra pay, I held my ground. Not long after I said 'no', I arrived at the office. Only a few people were there. "Don't worry, you just keep working," the team manager told me. Little did I know the others were meeting to discuss what to do about me, because I had said 'no' to the big boss. He wasn't happy, but he couldn't fire me because of Australia's unfair dismissal laws. So he was trying to see if I had botched any projects or made other mistakes for which he could dismiss me. He never found a cause. Colleagues vouched for me, and my record showed a steady string of going beyond the call of duty. I showed up, and it paid dividends.

Was I afraid to lose my job? Sure, but I was willing to take that risk. What I *was not* willing to do was to be treated as if I was just another number. I work hard, and I expect to be paid accordingly. As it turned out, I kept my job, and they hired another person to fill the vacant position. Ironically, a few months later I was offered a promotion to a position on the stock floor, with a higher salary attached.

Being loyal is about respecting yourself while doing your best, and about putting forth your top effort every day. It is *not* about compromising your principles or sense of fairness when someone tries to take advantage of you. Even your boss. This is a good way to minimize the stress surrounding your livelihood and long-range future.

Making the Company Goals Important to You

Along with loyalty comes buy-in. Every company sets targets and goals they want to accomplish. You need to be willing to get on board with those goals, with an attitude that you will do everything in your job description (and beyond) to help them achieve their objectives.

Work for your own fulfillment and feeling of self-worth, as well as the company's objectives. Find ways to become motivated and inspired enough to bring out your A game, and perform consistently at that level.

In my clinic, I help my clients return to their own dreams, desires and goals, so they can see what inspired and motivated them–and what might light those all-important fires again. So let's carry that simple exercise into this book:

Go back to the things that you really want in life. Ask yourself, "How is working with this company helping me achieve those goals?" Think of at least ten ways achieving the company goal will help you meet *your* goals.

Create rewards for yourself. As you accomplish targets, or mileposts, set by the company, give yourself a small reward. Likewise, as you move toward or accomplish your own goals, whether as part of your job or separately, reward yourself. For example, if one of your goals is to get a new car, and that is your motivation for achieving the set targets, then at the halfway mark, reward yourself with a fun event like a movie or something else you enjoy. Reward yourself so that you remain inspired to reach the company goals–and yours.

When you align your goals with the company's objectives, you find yourself highly motivated. The company's targets and objectives become a vehicle to achieving your own. This is especially evident in the academic field, in which you find tenured professors spending decades building curriculum and courses, and teaching students–but also writing books. How can they do both? Simple: their institutional goals grew into their personal goals, or vice-versa. From that came purpose-filled lives that benefitted others.

One thing to remember, however, is that the company is in business and the marketplace for itself. The executives and decision-makers are watching the good of the company, while you are ultimately trying to hit your goals. By helping them achieve their goals, they in turn help you achieve yours. You help them gain new customers and keep existing customers happy. In turn, they pay your salary, commissions and incentives, as well as support and subsidize training programs or seminars that add to your skills. These compensations help you achieve your goal.

Certainly, the stress levels in your life will be lower if you figure out how to meet your goals as you help the company achieve theirs, rather than always fighting against the current every time you show up for work.

The Team

We have probably all heard the little acronyms of TEAM: Together Everyone Achieves More. Or, Together Everyone Achieves Miracles. On a good team, everyone fulfills their part efficiently and effectively for the betterment of everyone involved.

A great team relies on every member's efforts to function and succeed. As a young child, I was a goalkeeper in soccer. I belonged to a very good and organized team that kept opponents out of our end of the pitch with teamwork, by playing together. I didn't have to do much at all. In fact, it could get very boring just standing in the box, more of a spectator than a player. On other occasions, when my team was not functioning well, I had my work cut out for me. I had to dive all over the place to stop goals.

Like any other sport, the aim of every soccer team is to win. Your backs need to do their job by keeping the ball at the other end, your midfielders need to control the tempo of the game, and your forwards need to put the ball in the back of the net. Finally, the goalkeeper must stop all opponents' shots for goals if opponents manage get past the backs. A well-trained and performing team will work together. How many sides have won the FIFA World Cup, Super Bowl, or NBA title against teams filled with superstars? Many more than you might think. Great teams consistently outperform teams of great individuals. To give another illustration, if you look at a watch, you might think a simple screw doesn't look that nice or important. So you discard it, cast it to the sideline. When you try to use the watch, it no longer functions.

Every good CEO and manager understands the importance of teamwork. They don't just dictate how and what it will happen, but work with the whole team, with each individual an integral part. Players get involved in the decision-making process and goal setting.

When I was studying, I worked part time at a factory doing freight handling for a courier company. I almost lost my hand when it was caught in a conveyor belt. Luckily for me, I managed to pull it out before a box full of bolts and screws rolled over it. All I suffered was an intense friction burn. I honestly thought I was going to lose my hand.

While doing all the first aid things necessary for my hand injury, I was sitting outside the office, and listening to the site manager–the number one man in the area. He was reminding one of the middle managers that everyone on the team was vital for the company to function. The middle manager countered by saying that he was better and more important than the others because of his place as a manager.

Why were the two talking? Because the middle manager had treated one of the freight handlers badly in the way he spoke and dealt with him. That freight handler couldn't take it anymore, and went to higher management. The higher manager pointed out that everyone was important and played a vital part, and each person needed to feel appreciated, or else they would leave, and the company would become that much weaker as a result. The middle manager's reply? The company could just hire someone else.

The site manager responded by saying that would cost money and time in training. It would also cause friction with other workers. That would reduce morale, and the team might not function properly. "Customers might stop doing business with us, and we are all out of a job. So it is better to just treat them well in the first place. Now, go and apologize and treat them well," the site manager concluded.

His comments really surprised me–in a good way. As I listened to the middle manager, I had thought that all managers in this company would be rude and uncaring about their workers. Then, when the higher manager spoke, I heard a different story. Higher managers (at least this one) actually cared about the workers, and were trying to help the middle managers see that lower-level workers were just as important to the company's overall success.

Make your relationship with your team stronger, and create higher performance and less stress in your workplace. Go back to your goals and align them with the team so that you are enlightened and energized. If you do this, and communicate and work well with your coworkers, you will be better able to do your best every time.

Taking Breaks

Quick breaks help you remain on top of your game. Give yourself little breaks, like going to the office kitchen and getting something to eat or drink, or walking outside for five minutes for fresh air. Stretch in the corner of your office, or take a little breather to quickly relax. When we take these little breaks, we rejuvenate ourselves and focus better. Our stress levels drop and we reenergize. The key to creating a low-stress environment is to use breaks as mini-rewards: "If I work hard on this report for the next hour, I'm taking a ten-minute break outside."

While getting my business up and running, I did some door-to-door sales for a company that set a daily goal of closing a certain number of sales. Each person was meant to achieve a fair percentage of the team's target. It was pretty hard going, but I would just keep going until I reached my target. If I didn't hit it, then I didn't get a break. I started to get discouraged after many days without hitting my goal–or taking a break. It became exhausting, counterproductive.

I decided to reward myself with a break when I reached the halfway mark to my target. I sat down, ate something quickly, and asked myself how this was helping me achieve my personal goals. After a twenty-minute break, I started up again. The little break helped me re-focus. I had rested, taken some time for myself, and focused on my goals. It made me happy to get up and sell again. It didn't feel like drudgery anymore.

In another part of my life, I worked with a colleague in the city. He would walk into the kitchen and not even get himself a coffee or something to eat, but he would perform some quick stretches for about five minutes. He would then return to his desk and start working again, feeling refreshed and energized. During his one-hour lunch break, rather than sit in a café, he would change into running gear and jog for twenty minutes. He would return, take a quick shower, get back in his work clothes and *then* find something to eat. When his lunch break ended, he was primed for a highly positive and productive afternoon.

Most people are highly productive in the morning, but less so after lunch. Why? Because they are tired or digesting big lunches. The body's natural rhythm runs on higher energy levels in the early morning and late afternoon hours than during the middle of the day; that's why the concept of siestas and the two-hour lunch breaks in most European Union countries took hold. However, my colleague was just as productive, or even more so, in the early afternoon than in the morning. He counteracted his body's feeling of fatigue by getting the blood pumping. He rejuvenated himself. Eventually, he became a manager. He encouraged his team to join him at lunch. Consequently, his section performed better than every other team in the second half of the day. They also felt a lot less stress.

When you have a short break, get the blood pumping and your brain moving again. That way, you stay motivated, rejuvenated and ready to work at peak efficiency, all of which feel very gratifying and purposeful. And you have less stress.

The Destructive Power of Gossip

Perhaps nothing causes more personal hurt, destroys team chemistry, damages reputations, or creates greater stress on the job than gossip. Of all the things that can ruin workplace morale, gossip ranks at or near the top. It's so preventable: all it takes is a closed mouth and a focus on minding our own business.

Why do people gossip? To push away real or imagined lacks in their lives by focusing on what they perceive to be troubles in the lives of others – and then spreading the "news" to draw attention to themselves. Gossip shows a lack of self-worth, a lack of purpose, and a lack of respect. People gossip out of jealousy over something they admire in another person that they don't see within themselves. They try to tear someone down to feel better, because they feel a lack of self-worth. The lower their opinion of themselves, the more they will gossip (if they are inclined to do so).

Most people who backstab or gossip are trying to build themselves up by convincing themselves that they are worth more–and their target is worth less. This may work for the short term, but not for any longer period. We all know what we think of ourselves deep down.

Another sad thing is that the gossipers are amazing in their own right. They don't need to tear others down to make themselves look better. Often, they are already great. Problem is, they don't see this, which is why they resort to gossip. To solve any urges to gossip, follow the steps in Chapter 8. When you have a healthy respect for yourself, you *won't want* to gossip. Even when things are frustrating and you feel like gossiping, you can decide not to. Gossip doesn't solve anything, but only creates further problems, so why do it?

I worked at a take away store while in high school. A bell went off whenever a customer came through the door. For some reason, I wanted to know if it was because of a sensor in the floor. One day, I ran over the spot that sets off the alarm, and the bell didn't ring. To my surprise, it didn't tell me anything. So I went around the back to check my roster. As I checked, I heard the managers and all but one staff member talking about a co-worker. When I realized their backstabbing was directed at me, I couldn't help but join in. We carried on this great conversation about how bad I was, and no one even noticed until another staff member walked in. I was having as much fun as anyone gossiping about myself! As soon as they realized I was there, they turned around and said they were joking. I told them I knew they weren't. I didn't really care, because I worked only to get paid. That was it. I did point out, "Don't worry, you get gossiped about when you're not here as well". They replied very defensively that they did not talk about each other. So I polled every single person in the room as to their comments about others. A big argument erupted over what they had said about each other. I checked my roster and left while they continued their heated argument.

If you gossip about others, chances are good that they are saying the same types of things about you. Often, those with whom you gossip are often the culprits who are against you! They will rarely admit it, but here's the thing: if someone gossips with you present, why wouldn't they gossip when you are absent? A gossip is a gossip, a person looking for an audience.

There are two ways to look at gossip. You can get upset and angry that they are talking about you, which will simply add to the stress in your life and fulfill their objective–to lift themselves up while bothering you, putting you down. Or, you can say, "I am so important to them that they talk about me." No matter how hurtful their comments, you will find it hard to get upset when you see it from this perspective. You can also build your self-confidence with the steps in Chapter 8.

Another thing to point out: what others think of you is really none of your business. It doesn't matter if their opinion is good or bad. Live the way you want, regardless. If others don't like that, it has nothing to do with you. Rather, it reflects their insecurities and their baggage.

In the workplace–or any other place, for that matter–gossip destroys. It destroys morale, productivity, teamwork, and cooperation. It consumes anything around it, hurts the team's efforts to be productive and move forward, and impedes your progress to meet your goals. The best advice? Ignore it and steer clear. Don't add to it.

Still Battling Peer Pressure

Remember peer pressure from the schoolyard and classroom? We felt it from all sides when growing up, and it served as a character builder–whether or not we saw it that way. Then, when we became adults, it dropped from our lives permanently, like baby teeth ... right?

Not necessarily. The truth is that as long as you have peers, you will circle the vicinity of peer pressure. It is a lifelong presence. Your peers surround you at work, group activities, or on sports teams if you still compete. The reality is, you were not friends with every single person in your class, but they are still considered your peers. Sometimes, the ones with whom we barely communicated are those who tried to pressure us into doing something that we didn't want to do.

Peer pressure can actually be a good thing, because when it happens, you have to make decisions. Usually, our peers would encourage us to try things like cigarettes, drugs and alcohol, skipping school, or other mischievous acts (or worse) that would not help our lives. For example, when I talk or work with smokers, I ask them how they started. Often, they first lit up at school–to gain acceptance from their peers. What was it like? I ask. They said they would cough, and feel choked up, or didn't like the taste. They continued to smoke only to fit in with their friends.

This is the face of peer pressure we most often see. The flip side is something much different, what I call peer support. In this case, peers encourage us to do things that improve our lives or skills, increase our potential, and help us perform better. Some of these acts include studying hard, practicing regularly in sport, art, musical or other activities, and developing the courage to go for it in life.

What about in the workplace? Whether you realize it or not, your colleagues are your peers. Sometimes, they may try to pressure you into doing something that you shouldn't do or don't want to do. Just as in school, this can cause great stress and trauma. Even little taunts or dares can cause stress. These can range from stealing a pen from the office to spiking someone's coffee with enough sugar to overdose an elephant. It gets bad when it becomes criminal, like embezzling large sums of money. Either way, you know that you shouldn't be doing it. You have to make the decision whether or not to move forward. If you bow to the dare and take a negative action, you are not being true to yourself.

Now let's look at some of the benefits. First, you learn the limits of what you are willing to accept. You can improve your strength in making choices of your own, and for yourself. You can also better understand that you are unique and distinct from any other person. Peer pressure can teach you better negotiation skills. As you negotiate with your peers, you can master the skills needed for a job interview or pay rise.

The positive side of peer pressure can also introduce you to things you may never have liked before–or never thought of at all–such as different types of music, sports, art and other new experiences. It can also help you to find worthwhile activities, like working with youth or a charity. As you involve yourself with these new, positive experiences, you build confidence from learning new skills or from meeting new people. It can help you push yourself beyond your comfort zone to take calculated risks, and see things from a new perspective. Think of someone who is afraid to run again after suffering a broken hip, then joins her spouse in his running group. She intends to walk, but when she sees the other ten people jogging, she joins them for the first mile–and finds out she can run. The "pressure" came from watching ten highly positive people run, and wanting to join in. That's a positive result.

How do you deal with peer pressure? First, decide if you are being true to yourself. Are you being true to your goals, dreams, values and beliefs? Is it something that will help you or others? Do you want to do it? If so, then go with it. If not, who is gaining the benefit? You? Or the other person? If you do what they ask, is it carrying you toward or away from your goals and dreams? Will you feel better about yourself–or worse? These questions will help you decide. If you have given into peer pressure and feel guilty about it, learn from past mistakes. Stand on your own two feet, so that the mistake becomes a learning experience rather than a regret.

There are different skills that will help you if you don't want to act on something that others are pressuring you to do. The first is assertiveness. Return to your goals, and see if the other's request will help you attain them. If not, learn to say "No". It is a beautiful, liberating two-letter word when used correctly. If you're still not sure how to deal with peer pressure, find someone you trust and seek their advice. This doesn't mean you will act on what they say, but their counsel can benefit you.

Finally, help yourself deal with peer pressure by making the decision beforehand. When I was younger, I already knew that cigarettes, alcohol, and drugs were not good for me, so I chose not to try them before anyone even approached me. I didn't want to end up like some of my friends, who chose to use these things in their lives, just because they tried to persuade me to give it a go.

Love Working

When you choose a career you love, it minimizes some or even most of the stress you feel in the workplace. In talking with clients and people, I have learned that most people find it hard to be inspired, even when they are pursuing their goals and dreams. Most said they are only working at the best job they can find or one that allows them to afford a certain lifestyle, rather than undertaking the type of work they really want. They settle for what pays the bills instead of what pleases their hearts, minds and souls.

Here is a large-scale example of how working at what you love minimizes stress, no matter the workload. When he was a penniless 24-year-old musician, Stevie Salas dropped into the opportunity of a lifetime: playing lead guitar on Rod Stewart's 1988-89 Out of Order World Tour. The gig seemed way over his head, but he believed in himself, because he loved what he was doing and was good at it. Stevie literally went from playing local backyards to center stage at the world's largest stadiums in three years! He later toured with Mick Jagger, Duran Duran and Terence Trent d'Arby as well. Still, the touring life with superstar bands didn't fulfill him–though most of us would think, "Are you crazy? That's the dream of millions!"

Stevie then struck career gold doing something he loves: producing albums, writing songs and working on TV and movie projects. While touring with his own bands, Stevie went on to produce, perform and record more than 90 albums–10 of them his own. He knows or has played with virtually every major musician of the past 40 years. He's been musical director on *American Idol,* the music advisor to the Smithsonian Institution, and is now a film and television producer while continuing as a recording artist. The man works long hours routinely while jetting from Toronto to Montreal, to Washington D.C. to Chicago, to Los Angeles to his Texas home.

But here's the thing: he's always smiling, talkative, and guaranteed to light up a room with his personality and positive attitude. When he talks about his work, he *brings it*–the enthusiasm, joy, and fascination with being in the same workspace as our favorite music superstars. Why? Because everything he does revolves around music, his favorite thing in the world. He has helped countless musicians, put out great music of his own, and become very successful by being a "go to" guy. In case you're wondering, 25 years after touring with Rod Stewart, he still gets a taste of the old star treatment: fans in Europe and Japan consider him a superstar. When you love your work, it doesn't feel like work. It adds to the joy of life, which diminishes stress.

Many of my clients have walked into job interviews, attracted by an advertisement that said the starting salary would fall between A and B. They opted for A, because it was the lower amount. They thought their chances of landing the job were higher if they sought the lower pay. In my talks with many employers, they always tell me they prefer candidates who opt for the higher amount and then negotiate, because they look at those asking for lower pay as less skilled, qualified or confident.

One of my clients started off working in a factory. He honestly thought himself only good enough for this type of job. He took many different courses to learn different machines and tools so he could progress on the factory floor. Through a series of events, many sales reps were let go. One of the managers liked my client, and asked if he would like to move into sales. My client didn't think he could do it, but after the manager reassured him that his old job would be waiting if the sales position didn't work out, he agreed to switch. The new position would increase his salary from thirty thousand to sixty thousand dollars a year, plus bonuses. However, he remained scared, because he had never tried sales and didn't know if he could do it. He didn't even like working in the factory.

This story has a happy ending. He performed extremely well, and he enjoyed his work much more than the factory floor. Because he was doing so well, several competitors tried to poach him. Many were even willing to double his *new* salary–into the $120,000 range. His company further recognized his value, and gave him a big pay rise and a company car.

What a difference an opportunity makes! Before, he settled for what he thought his potential to be. However, when the opportunity came and he took it, his whole life changed. Choose something you love so that you *want* to go to work.

Another client worked in a telecom company as a technician, but loved talking to people and helping them. Word got back to the managers of how happy customers were when they spoke to him. His boss understood the man's greater value, and offered him a position in customer service and relations.

At first, my client wasn't sure about the new position, but decided to go for it. He didn't even have the same guarantee to return to his old job as the first example. As it turned out, he didn't need a safety net at all. His pay went up, he loved his new responsibilities, and he helped the business grow. He was much happier with working and felt much less stress because he enjoyed it. Eventually, he left the company and started his own business, and succeeded handsomely. He became more inspired because he learned to go for what he wanted by trying something new.

If you want to be inspired in your work, then choose something you love. Choose something that utilizes your natural strengths. When you do this, work transforms into a form of play. At least it feels like play. When companies, clients or others see you excelling at something you thoroughly enjoy, they will be drawn to your energy as if you were a magnet. Prosper–and have fun doing it.

Magnify to Simplify

To magnify is to make something appear larger than it really is, especially with a lens or microscope. To simplify is to make something easier to do or understand. How do these two come together in your workplace and career?

If we magnify a cell under a microscope, we see and better understand its properties. The naked eye can't come close to seeing the activity. We cannot understand it without a magnifying instrument. Now, we can break down its many processes into simple, easy-to-understand parts. We simplify and improve our ability to study the cell by magnifying it.

How does this concept apply to the workplace? Often, people magnify the impact of their job on their lives and health by doing far more than necessary, or making it look harder by not being organized for effectiveness and efficiency. In this instance, we need to break it into smaller parts (simplify) to be more effective (magnify). We simplify how much and what we are doing, but magnify the effect, achieving better results from the same amount of effort. What makes us most effective at work, performing to our highest capabilities without feeling stressed out and hurting our performance? Simplifying, and achieving maximum results.

When we become more efficient and smart about doing our jobs, we do not have to work as hard, or as long, to get the same effect, impact and result. Less work carries less stress; we don't have to cram as much into the day. Complication equals more stress, while simplification equals more peace.

I gain a lot of insight from checking out the appearance of a work desk. How organized is the person? Do they value order? Is their life stressful, or tranquil? If you have a messy desk, it can be difficult to find the things that you need, and take longer because you have to sift through more piles. Over a day, or a week, this costs enough of your time that deadlines become harder to meet, magnifying the amount of work to be done.

What gets lost? Your effectiveness. You are now doing more work to achieve the same result, which equals more stress. If the desk were organized in the first place, you would be more proficient, and meet deadlines more easily while causing yourself less stress.

A good example of this is an experience I had concerning a rubber stamp and stickers. I was handwriting addresses on envelopes for a mailer, a process that took at least half an hour, making it hard to beat the postman's deadline. When I started using the return address stamp, it more than reduced the time needed by 50% when filling out those envelopes. Then, when I received the address stickers for the intended recipients, it only took about five minutes to complete a job that took more than half an hour before. I simplified my efforts while magnifying my result. Do you think a spare twenty-five minutes minimized my stress levels? Of course. This solution also made it easier for many people in the office when they posted a large amount of mail.

Job Security

The question of job security stresses out many people. We look for security within our jobs, finances, relationships, houses, possessions and so on. Problem is, we always look for it *out there*.

Really, our security comes from within us. It is the quiet self-confidence and self-assurance that we will be OK, no matter the situation, because of our skills and knowledge of how to move forward.

To measure such things, businesses use a SWOT analysis form–Strengths, Weaknesses, Opportunities, and Threats. We will review SWOT as it pertains to ourselves, not the companies we own or that employ us.

What are your STRENGTHS? Look at what you bring to the table, at what sets you apart from the competition and helps you to rise above it. Look at what you do in order to be more proficient and productive, and what gives you a competitive edge.

What are your WEAKNESSES? This step is hard for many people, because we tend to be extra harsh on ourselves when we fall short. Or, if we don't want to beat ourselves up, we tend to lightly brush over them. So here's a news flash that will help you feel better: *everyone* has weaknesses. Be rigorously honest about your weaknesses, without kicking yourself too hard. Identify, notice and face them. Do not brush over them, but see them instead as *opportunities to grow*. By acknowledging weaknesses, we start to convert them into strengths. The abilities you gain while improving yourself may directly help you be a better worker. Michael Jordan once said, "Always turn a negative situation into a positive situation." Look at your weaknesses, and see how you can turn them into a positive strength for yourself.

What are our OPPORTUNITIES? These weaknesses create opportunities to grow, strengthen, and do better. Recognizing opportunity is the ability to see the promise or potential in a person or situation, and using your strength, skill and determination to create the outcome you envision. Nothing is better material with which to work than your own weaknesses, because when you turn them into opportunities to improve, you greatly strengthen yourself. Opportunities also come from our effectiveness, including the chance to learn new skills and become a bigger asset to the company.

Finally, what are the THREATS? Often, they are your perceived weaknesses. Where do you always fall short? How does it continue to impact your life? Work on these areas. Another great threat to our wellbeing comes when we "rest on our laurels," deciding that everything is fine and there is no need to become better than yesterday. That is a one-way ticket to lower job standing.

Politicians often resort to name calling or slinging mud at the other party. So often they are so focused on slinging the mud that they do not focus on the good they could bring to their countries. Eventually, the general population gets fed up and disillusioned, because politicians choose not to pass legislation to solve their problems. When it comes time to vote, we feel like we're choosing between the lesser of two losers to lead the country. Or, worse, that our opinion doesn't count at all. If politicians focused more on what they could do for their country, both they and the people would move forward.

Instead of thinking about tearing down and bringing out the worst in each other to keep our job security, instead focus on your performance, strengths and what you can add in a particular position. If you tear someone else down, you reveal your own insecurity. If you talk about your strengths and vision, then your manager or director will already know what unique and distinct qualities you bring to the position. *That* is job security.

Competition

Competition is a big dynamic and perhaps a bigger issue in the workplace. First, you size up the situation. Who is your competition? Other companies? Divisions? The person sitting next to you? Next, you strategize ways to beat them. Some people are more competitive than others, but the key to reducing workplace stress is to find ways to channel competitive people into winning contracts and the like, while moving less competitive people into supportive but equally important roles in servicing those contracts. Competition can define, build or disrupt an organization. It can help or hinder your life, either taking you further or slowing you down with too much stress.

Start by looking at yourself. If you're an average employee, then everyone is your competition. Anyone who wants your job can be considered competition, as can anyone who holds the job you seek. This is often the scenario people consider when they refer to the "dog eat dog world", because you and the other person see each other as competition in a tough game of "survival of the fittest".

How do you set yourself apart? How do you rise above the competition without resorting to cutthroat techniques that might get you the position, but cost you friends and respect in the process? First, work out what is unique about yourself. What do you bring to the table that distinguishes you? Speed? Efficiency? A particular talent? The way you make customers feel at ease? Answering these and other similar questions will assist you in setting yourself apart from, and then rising above, your competition.

The next thing is to realize that your greatest competition is *you*. Often, we hear great sports champions say something like, "I'm not worried about what the other team is going to do. I'm worried about whether I can do everything in my power to win this game." You name a great sports figure, and I guarantee you this is how they think. If you can win the competition within yourself, and continuously push yourself to higher levels, then how much do you really need to worry about the opponent?

Your competition is who you were yesterday. Are you doing better? Are you being more effective? Are you accomplishing more today than yesterday? When you ask and answer these questions, you will learn if you are beating your real competition or not. As a general rule, if you can improve every day, or at least know you did your best, then you will rise above any real or perceived competition.

The big problem we face isn't competition at all. It's *complacency*. Often, we get so comfortable with our current station that we do the bare minimum to pick up our pay check. When we allow ourselves to become complacent, we become prime targets for others who want our jobs. If we want to stay ahead, then we continue to work at being better today than we were yesterday. It is more fulfilling, and reduces unneeded stress.

Keeping Educated

One way to have more security and rise above any perceived competition is to upgrade your skills and keep educated. Keep up to date with what is new in your field, and keep educating yourself. For starters, you can use the SWOT analysis to determine the areas in which more education will strengthen your hand and lead to greater opportunities. Think of the man early in the chapter, who moved from the factory floor to the sales line. Along the way, he had to educate himself in an entirely new area. He accepted the challenge, and emerged with a very rewarding career.

Those who keep their minds active through education, reading, word games and other activities age slower than those who don't. It's not only a benefit for your career, but for your health as well. Start now. Two men that I know are on the older side of life. One of them is in his sixties and he walks around like a little old cripple with his walking frame. The other man is well into his eighties, yet he walks around more like a healthy fifty year old.

Education doesn't have to be in a classroom, university, college, or any other formal school. In fact, often universities and colleges are often behind, as technology and research are moving forward too fast for them to respond. Some universities make slow, lumbering turns like ocean cruise liners, but unfortunately, we live in a test pilot world where we often have to turn on a dime and switch directions instantly.

While university is very important coming out of prep or high school years, its role diminishes as you get older, depending on your career of choice. By the time a new text is printed, research and knowledge has come forward to outdate the content. I know a college professor in California who teaches online communications by gathering white papers before each quarter, copying them onto flash drives, and handing flash drives to students–with links to keep updated. That assures up-to-the-minute education. You can read books, conduct research on the Internet, or listen to inspirational people and audio books. You can talk to other people in the industry.

Continually educate yourself in your field, or one you wish to enter. Become a leader of yourself. You will have more to give. This gives you a competitive edge and more security within, leading to more job security and less stress.

Dealing With The Bully

Do you remember walking across the schoolyard, your heart pumping, paranoid eyes scanning the grounds, hoping that the school bully wasn't waiting for you? Remember holding that fear of being threatened out of your school lunch money, or punched because the guy felt like hitting someone? Or how you wondered, "Why is he (or she) picking on me?" and questioning why bullies were allowed to breathe at all?

Perhaps this situation is too familiar, even now. You are at work, you go about your day, fulfilling your role, doing your job. All of a sudden, crisis strikes. Like a tornado, a co-worker confronts you over some discrepancy. She takes it further than simply demanding better job performance; she shreds you to pieces. Your sense of credibility and confidence shrink to zero. After the event, resentment stews in you like the caldera at Kilauea. You imagine scenarios in which you verbally high-five your accoster's face, smacking him or her down with one comeback after another. You can't focus on work; after all, this insensitive co-worker or supervisor has ruined your day!

Why do people bully each other? Why do they make another's life miserable–and then repeat the act until someone stands up to the offender? When we are kids, bullies look like monsters in human form. As we get older, we learn something that is surprising at first, then seemingly the most obvious thing–bullies are insecure. Maybe they were bullied themselves, and try to take out their pain and anger on others. A bully will only harass someone over which they feel they have power. If they do not view themselves having the upper hand, they will not even try.

There are two types of bullies: the schoolyard bully who is physically aggressive; and the verbal bully. The latter is of big concern in the workplace. The verbal bully operates with threats, raised voices, lying, gossiping and backstabbing. They can be sneaky, passive aggressive types, setting you up to get fired or smearing egg on your face. They will say things or put you in positions to look bad. If you let them emotionally affect you, they eventually succeed, diminishing your effectiveness and causing self-doubt and stress.

There are ways to confront bullying–and I do mean CONFRONT. However, they do not involve stooping to the bully's level of stupidity and insecurity. If you do, and someone walks past during a confrontation, the passerby won't be able to distinguish the aggressor. Many bullies are quick to portray you as the aggressor, because that is what they do well. They have years of practice. Needless to say, your stress levels spike in these situations.

Don't stoop to their level. Confront them and point out why they are acting out in the first place. Encourage them to stop. Do this in a way where you are covered legally and professionally.

One of my clients was a registered nurse working in a hospital. She would pick up a colleague from the train station and drive him to work. This colleague was a self-appointed manager. Many of the woman's colleagues and patients loved and respected her, because she was hard working and caring to everyone, patients and co-workers alike.

However, the self-appointed manager was afraid of her. He feared her potential. He worried she would move up the ranks quickly and take the position to which he aspired. So he started to attack her, going so far as to fraudulently fill out legal documents to make it look as though she was not doing her job. Instead of going to my client to tell her he thought she missed something, he complained to higher management, to make her look incompetent. He proceeded directly to the CEO, and explained how and why she was unsatisfactory.

Then the bullying started–from the guy she kindly picked up from the station!

At first, her situation grew worse. She had the courage to confront the bully, as well as her manager, who was briefed by the CEO. Both were friends of her accuser. The manager downplayed the fact the man had fraudulently filled out and signed off on these legal documents. Her stress levels rose so much that she could not do her job. She couldn't think properly. The hospital sent her to its psychologist–another friend of the manager's. Eventually, she sought legal advice on how to sort out the problem.

When she came to me for help, she had been declared unfit to work for two months. In our first session, we found clarity over what was happening, why it was happening, how she was dealing with it, and what she needed to do. She had been bullied many times earlier in her life. She did not stop it then, or now, for the same reason–she lacked assertiveness skills and the ability to recognize when someone was pulling a dirty one on her. This made her vulnerable to the full attack that followed.

As part of the process, she let go of some of her past pain and her deep fears about being assertive. She then learned ways of being assertive in this specific situation, and felt confident enough to tackle work again.

She returned to the company-appointed psychologist, who was amazed at how much more clear and unstressed she seemed. However, he was unhappy that the things that he had been doing to her no longer kept her feeling stuck and helpless, (remember: again, he was a friend of the manager's, who was in turn a friend of the bully).

She came back for her second appointment with me; afterwards, she was cleared to work again. When she returned, word had funneled to management that she had stood up to the psychologist. The bully and manager stayed away from her. They saw she was unafraid of dealing with them, and realized she could have them jailed for fraud or harassment. She never had a problem with them again. Better yet, within a few months, she took a new job in a more positive environment. As for the bully? Ironically, he suffered a heart attack just before she switched jobs. One insecure person caused all of this turmoil and stress, but it was complicated by her lack of empowerment in dealing with him.

Bullies act out because they fear something great they see within you. This can range from your potential to what you are already accomplishing... and sometimes, even from what you *won't* do. In most cases, directly dealing with the bully can help. If you do, never put them in position where they risk losing face; that will worsen the situation. When sorting it out with the bully doesn't work, go to the manager. If this does not work, you may need to seek legal aid.

One of the things that has helped many of my clients in bullying situations is to point out their own insecurity. You may not know the exact cause, but you know the person is insecure. If you address it, sometimes that alone will prompt them to stop and think about their own issues, rather than focusing on your psyche.

In this and every workplace situation, the ball circles back to a recurring theme: has this happened before in your life? And how does the situation help you now, and in the future? How are you growing from the experience? Sometimes, you may need to change your job, or find ways to reduce your stress within the workplace. If you don't deal with a stress-inducing work situation, it will return in various shapes and sizes–or people–until you have figured out how to work with it.

Chapter 7: Your Money or Your Life: Stress and Finances

How many times have our otherwise great days or weeks come crashing down because of finances? Either we don't have enough money, or we over-spend into a financial crunch. Even worse, we may load ourselves up with enough credit card debt to sink our loftiest dreams. When we turn 40, 50 or 60, and realize that our fun-loving, free spending ways have hurt our long-held retirement goals, what happens? We suffer from the resulting stress, sometimes in the form of chronic ailments.

Not a pretty picture, is it? The problems become more stressful and debilitating when we look at them in terms of relationships. While one partner lives conservatively, doing her part to save money, the other lives like a high roller. When the housing market and economy drop out, home values and retirement plans tumble as well, entirely out of your control. Maybe you didn't make enough salary, or put enough of it away. Perhaps your planning didn't take into account those hidden expenses, changes in economic fortunes, or the fact that tuition for your 6-year-old will be three times higher than you originally budgeted for.

When financial difficulty rears its ugly head, our happiness and peace of mind suffer. Our stress levels automatically rise – a lot. Our ability to love and nurture our partners properly diminishes. The cortisol levels in our brain spike until all we can see in our frantic tunnel vision are two options - fight or flight. We blame the system. We blame our boss. We blame the money-based economy. We blame our partners. We beat ourselves up. We stop loving and respecting ourselves. All for something as neutral and lifeless on its own as the currency you hold in your hand.

Yes, finances are a central and necessary part of life. Money does contribute to the type of lifestyle we choose and the plans we make. Most of us do attach a measure of self-worth, satisfaction and happiness to the amount of money we make. And yes, our financial situation leads to more or less stress, depending on its status.

Rather than run from the obvious, stressing ourselves out some more, I recommend we tackle this issue directly. By gaining control over our financial situations, and using them to work *in our favor,* we can deal with one of the greatest sources of stress in our lives. When we do that, we alleviate the stress – especially when we maintain focus and consistency over our financial matters. These issues can be solved in three ways:

1. Practical steps to improve the financial situation
2. Looking into the reasons for the thought processes behind the behavior
3. Correcting the thought processes

These three steps can help you overcome financial stress and enjoy more success. In many cases, just changing habits or taking practical steps is enough. But in many others, you need more. You may not possess the self-discipline to take all of the steps. You may start with the right intentions and focus, but then give up somewhere along the way. That creates more stress and casts self-doubt. Unfortunately, when dealing with issues like financial troubles or relationship dynamics, self-doubt doesn't just go away. It becomes layered with the next failed attempt, and the next, until you believe there is nothing you can do to resolve your difficulties. That piles on greater, more paralyzing stress. Let's approach our relationship with finances from the beginning – when we were too young to know anything more about money than the allowances our parents gave us.

Who Did You Learn From?

Think about the person from whom you learned your money management skills. Was it a parent? Loved one? Friend? Mentor? Call that person to mind. Now, think about how that person contributed to your approach to finances. Try to remember exactly what they told you, and connect their advice to specific aspects of your financial picture. Are you investing like Grandpa said? Are you saving at the percentage of income Uncle Tom suggested? Are you cutting corners on household expenses the way Mom taught you?

Go further back, and look at the results they have achieved (or fallen short on) in their lives. Are they living blissfully within their financial circumstances, or are they stressed because of them? Are they content? Comfortable? How are your results similar to these? How are they different? Are these the results you really want?

Answer these questions openly and honestly. Once you do, and have worked out whom you are emulating, you are in a position to set some goals. If the person you have been modeling yourself after is achieving the results you want, then build on that and keep going. What else are they doing? What more do you need to be doing that maybe they cannot teach you? Set goals around these types of questions.

Next, take a further step: how can I save better or more? How do I invest my money better? What can I do for a more fulfilling life, financially? Dig deeper. Set your goals around the answers. The more specific and defined the goal, the more likely you are to achieve it.

However, if the person from whom you learned is falling short of the results that you want – or has fallen short – ask yourself: Am I seeing those same results by following their example? If so, then you need to find someone else from whom to learn, or take it upon yourself to become more educated in finance and more frugal in your spending habits.

Here's an example. John, a young construction contractor, grew up in a household with two free-spending parents. His Mom even made a joke of bills that arrived in the post: "If the envelope has a window, throw it back." More than a few times, she wrote "recipient unknown" on the envelopes! While Mom spent everything in sight, and ran up massive credit card debts, Dad worked all day to bring in money–and had some expensive habits of his own. Both parents lost complete sight of *their parents'* financial habits, which involved careful spending, consistent saving, and smart investing.

By 17, John held down two jobs, while also pitching his high school baseball team to a championship and sporting a solid academic record. He had already squirreled away more than $5,000 in savings–an impressive feat for *any* 17-year-old. He grew tired of his parents borrowing money off him (once, even raiding his savings account without his knowledge!). He secretly started off his younger sisters with $500 bank accounts. Every time his parents asked for money, he rebuffed them–not because he didn't love them, but because he knew they would waste it. When they asked him how much he had, he said, "I'm broke." Then he opened an empty wallet. (While I do not like someone describing themselves as "broke", in this case, it was necessary.) Through years of watching his parents deal with debt collectors, repossessions and the like, he learned finances the hard way.

This happened years ago. Today, John is 30. He owns a small construction company, provides for his wife and three small kids, and pays cash for his "toys" – motorcycles, four-wheelers, and a small boat. His savings are in the low six figures, and his kids have college accounts, even though only the oldest is of kindergarten age.

How did John do it? How did he overcome his parents' negative financial practices to become a self-made success? He looked *beyond* them. He went to his grandparents, who were painfully aware of their children's financial woes (one grandfather even lost $10,000 on what he thought was a business loan to his son, funds that his daughter-in-law misappropriated for a shopping spree). He followed his grandparents' prudent financial example, and created a lifestyle far less stressful and more successful than his parents.

Look for someone around you, whether in person, over the Internet, or in a book. (If the latter, go with an author who is a recognized financial expert.) See how they are attaining the results that you want. Learn what they are doing. Learn how they are doing it. Then go through the steps I listed earlier. Set your new goals. They will free you to move forward. That feels uplifting and liberating, places of the mind where stress cannot lurk.

Achieving Balance

It's time to let go of illusions about our goals and living in balance. Now that we have started to set these goals, we need to give ourselves permission to dig deeper. First, write a Pros and Cons list to know and understand what you will need to do to achieve your goal. Here is an example about having the goal to be promoted to a management level position:

Pros:

1. Different style of work. More decision making, which I like, and fewer mundane tasks

2. Pay rise!

3. Opportunity to attract the attention of higher management, which could be good for further advancement

4. Gain professional skills that will help further my career

5. Get the credit and praise when things go well

Cons:

1. Dealing with disgruntled customers when they ask to speak to management
2. Dealing with more workplace dynamics if my team doesn't like my decisions or is envious of my progress
3. More accountability and responsibility to those that outrank me (I have to perform well, and take responsibility for problems my team members create)
4. Work more hours (occasionally)
5. Additional effort to learn needed skills

With many goals, the pros far outweigh the cons. In some situations, though, it may not be worth it. When I was 19, I was offered a promotion to learn stock broking on the trading floor. The training position started at $50,000 per year, a lot for a 19-year-old! However, I turned it down, despite the great financial benefit. From working in the stock broking industry, I had already seen that brokers worked incredibly long hours under high pressure. Many were burning out by age 30. I wanted a career that would last longer, and that I would enjoy more. I didn't take the promotion.

It's not always rosy and perfect. Look at people that seem to have it all–on the outside. While many are happy and fulfilled, others are not. They own big houses and expensive cars. Many tell us that they don't stay up at night stressing over something they can't afford. However, their stress might come from somewhere else, brought on by the same source: trying to afford a lifestyle. If they can afford it, are they living the way they really want? Are they *enjoying* that house or car? Or are they so busy stressing and working to maintain that lifestyle that they cannot enjoy it? There are two sides to everything.

Balance is about more than money. A wealthy person may be set financially, but his or her social life may be nonexistent. This dynamic is fine if they are workaholics and fulfill themselves entirely through work or investing, but otherwise… Now for the big question: would *you* enjoy being in that position? That needs to be taken into consideration. Ever wonder why many men in their 40s and 50s often revert to their teen years–surfing more than ever, growing their hair longer, buying speedy cars, trying to converse, in lingo, with teenagers? Because they focused so much on building a family and a nest egg, starting at a young age, that they gave up those necessary final growing-up years. Also, with the children out of the house, they can afford their toys.

Your values play a big part in goal setting. If you value family highly, you may not go out socializing. If you value socializing, you may not be willing to put in the needed time to start and run a business. If you value spiritual growth, you may not put in the time to look after your health–even though spiritual growth, health and well-being are truly part of the same process. Decide if you are willing to sacrifice core values in one area to feed another, and consider it when setting goals. Once you have gone through the Pros and Cons you can make a more informed decision as to what you want. Strike a balance.

A story along these lines: a man was doing well financially, but then decided he wanted to become a millionaire. After he made the decision, he achieved it. While setting the goal, he envisioned a lifestyle much better than he already had built for himself. However, even after he was earning up to three million dollars a year, he realized the new "lifestyle" wasn't all that he expected. He was working exceedingly long hours, sometimes seven days a week. He owned a nicer car and house, but had no life to speak of outside work.

One day, he looked at his life and didn't like what he saw. He reviewed his income and expenses, and realized he could live off $250,000 a year, including plenty of savings and charitable donations. He trimmed his workload and time spent on the job, and reclaimed his life. He made necessary changes, and now is a much happier man. He earns what he needs, while still enjoying the lifestyle he was chasing in the first place.

Budgeting and Filing

Now that we have decided what we want, and reviewed the Pros and Cons, we need to look at the "B" word. Budgeting. So many people want to earn big dollars and live fancy lifestyles, but they don't realize how self-made wealth was often created – by years of developing and following budgets with the discipline of a military officer. It's the day-after-day effort that creates success.

The first action in establishing a budget is to acknowledge your present position. Be rigorously honest. Are you in a financial surplus? Or a deficit? Maxed out with credit cards? Up to your eyeballs in car loans, home loans, business loans, personal loans, or any other type of loan? Or are you rolling in money, with loads to spare? Don't sugarcoat your situation with statements like, "Oh, we will be fine just the way it is." If you sugarcoat you will remain exactly where you are. Nothing wrong with that, of course, if it makes you happy. However, chances are, when you're forced to sit down and budget after years of not watching your money, debt and stress have rendered you something other than happy.

Set your limits. Look at the amount you spend–and what you spend it on. Set limits on the different areas of life and how much you can afford for each area. You would be surprised how money leaks from places we never consider. Several years ago, personal finance author David Bach (*Finish Rich*) coined a term: "the Latte Factor." This was based on the public's growing addiction to Starbucks coffee. If we add up the money we spend buying coffee or tea in coffeehouses, the totals might be staggering. Taken further, the Latte Factor applies to any way we spend little bits of money, repeatedly–downloading iTunes, shopping online, buying apps, feeding our book-buying habit on Amazon, getting a beer with the mates… or drinking lattes. The problem doesn't occur when we make these purchases. If they add to our life in some way, great! The problem, rather, is how *often* we buy–and how rarely these items show up in our family budgets. In America, for instance, it is considered normal for a businessman or woman to spend more than $40/week buying teas and coffees, one purchase at a time. Multiply that by 52 weeks, and you have nearly $2,100.

The first thing that I recommend to clients with maxed-out credit cards is to shred the card and make affordable payments to bring down the principal. With credit cards, there is a temptation to spend money you don't have. Removing that temptation makes it so much easier to stick to a budget. This is a hard decision for people used to living off the card, but a massive step towards having freedom and peace. As you consider this, ask yourself: why do I spend on credit cards? Why do I keep buying stuff? Is something missing in my life? Am I compensating for past or current lack in other areas of life? Why do I buy when stressed? How stressed out will I get from putting myself in this maxed-out position?

The next step? *Pay cash.* I thought I was pretty good at this, but when I committed to only use cash, I realized how often I was swiping my eftpos card. When I started paying with cash, I became pickier about what I would buy. Which leads to the next question: do I really need or want something enough to go to the bank to get the cash out? For me, the answer was often "No." Consequently, the money went towards something more important. Or, I saved it.

Using only cash can be a bit of a headache at first, because you need to remember to get the money. After that, you save money and keep it in your pocket. You work for your money. Now make it work for you. Keep it in your pocket, appreciate your own hard work in its green bill form, and watch your stress drop at the same time.

The next step is to file your receipts. This helps you see where you are spending your money. At the end of the month, you may look at your receipts and ask, "Did I really spend that much on my food?" or "I didn't realize that I was spending so much on going out and socializing." Figure out how you can cut that spending. "Do I really need to drive just around the corner, or can I just walk?" Don't get me wrong; it is very important to find a balance that gives you love, peace, joy and happiness. However, if you know how much and where your money is being spent, chances are you will improve your life standing.

As a kid, I was very frugal. I had a part time job and worked hard for that money. When I bought something, I didn't like seeing the money leave my hand. I always knew that I would earn more, but it was still a lot of effort. As I got older, swiping the card became easier and faster; I stopped thinking about how much I was spending. Now that I am back to cash, I watch how much I spend again.

Part of that comes from filing receipts. I file into ten categories, as shown me by my mentors, Robert Allen and Mark Victor Hansen:

1. Giving/Charity
2. Self
3. Taxes
4. Shelter
5. Household
6. Auto
7. Fun/Entertainment
8. Insurance
9. Debt/Miscellaneous
10. Business/Deductible Expenses

Once I started filing, I realized where I was spending money that I didn't need to spend. I looked for ways to save in those areas. Soon, I realized that I had more money than I'd thought.

Filing your receipts for a month or two may take a little time, but it can be a valuable wake up call. Another technique is to think about how much that pair of shoes would cost you after tax. Shopping psychologists advise retailers to cut off prices immediately below a whole number; say, $99.95 instead of $100. Studies have proven that sales increase for retailers who practice this pricing approach, because people think they are saving money. What happens when that $99.95 is taxed? If you are taxed at 20% off your income, and you buy a $99.95 pair of shoes, then you actually had to earn $124.95 for those shoes. What if you are taxed at 48%? Then it's almost a $200 pair of shoes.

Giving

An important step in becoming wealthy, or living a life with minimal financial stress, is donating to good causes. Many give 10% or more of their income to charity. This may seem strange to many who think the wealthy find any way possible to hold their money. The next thing many say? "It is just for tax benefits." Maybe so, but many wealthy people I have met gave charitably before they became wealthy. I am not saying that all the mega-rich practice this approach, but many do. To give an extreme example, the amount of money Bill and Melinda Gates have given through their philanthropic organization is higher than the gross national product (GNP) of some Third World countries.

I have introduced the concept of charitable giving to many clients. Some are skeptical at first, so I challenge them to live this way for one month, and then report back to me on how it helped them and how it felt. Many reported similar experiences: at first, they didn't really notice a difference in their personal finances, even though they were donating 10% of their income. Their money still seemed to stretch as far as before they made contributions. At the same time, they felt good within themselves (translation: unstressed). They paid their bills, put food on the table, and took care of their needs–and those of others. And often, their goal of giving more motivated them to take the steps needed to earn more. Nice.

There is a saying: "Givers get". Those willing to be generous will receive what they need. Then there's that other saying, "What goes around, comes around". This saying often implies something bad, but it works both ways. If you do unkind things, they will come back to you. If you do kind things, you will receive kindness in return. Those who are generous and kind are most likely to be rewarded generously. This does not necessarily mean financially, but financial reward is often a part of it.

Test this approach for yourself. Pick a charity that you like and feel good about, and give to it. I recommend you find one that puts a large percentage or even all donated funds into the cause itself (rather than admin costs). At the same time, continue taking your other budgeting steps. This is a great way to feel financial peace in your life.

Saving

The next step is to pay yourself. You may be thinking, "I just got paid by the company". Now, you are paying your savings account. So often, when the pay comes in, we look at all the bills and expenses and say, "I will pay all of these bills, and then save whatever is left". At the end, how much have you managed to save? Make saving a priority if you want to have financial peace in your life.

Many people have been taught that you have a particular amount of money, so this is how much you have to spend. Most people spend everything they have, with nothing left to save. There is always another thing to buy, or another sale, in which you buy something you didn't need and "save" on it. Or, you buy a discounted item, and then take the saved money to buy another item as you're waiting in checkout. Stores know this tendency very well; that is why most load up their point-of-purchase areas with tantalizing finger-sized items, magazines, candies, gift cards and the like.

Thirty to forty years ago, people lived off 80% to 90% of their income; the rest went into savings. Now, many live off *110%* of their income. When I speak to others about this, they make comments like, "Well, times are different now", or "But they were unhappy because they went without." Here's one that really strikes me: "You can't take your money with you, so you may as well enjoy it." One positive of the GFC, or great recession, is that more people are saving.

You have already paid 10% to a charity of your choice; now pay yourself 10% in an interest-bearing savings plan. It might start small, but it will grow over time. Not too long down the track, you may look at that account, and find an additional $10,000, to your surprise. All you did was put 10% aside, week after week–which inconvenienced you not at all. If you are saving for something particular, such as a house, car or holiday, you need to save for that in a separate savings account. This 10% account is for your financial future. By making these simple adjustments–10% to savings, 10% to charity–you are living off 80% of your income rather than 100%, plus whatever you were charging to credit cards. Chances are, you will discover that your lifestyle hasn't changed that much.

The only time you will start seeing an increase in financial peace is when you put these steps into action. Instead of little or no money in your account, you will start noticing increasingly higher numbers–and correspondingly lower amounts of stress.

Sacrificing and Keeping up with the Joneses

When we spend excessively, two reasons rise above all others: not having enough self-discipline; and trying to match the lifestyles of others. Ideally, we want happiness, and it need not require the biggest house, car or wardrobe to attain. It is best to make financial decisions from a logical point of view – "Do I need it?

Will it really improve my life?" – rather than an emotional state, where we only feel secure if we can compare favorably to the next highest economic level. That is a very fleeting form of happiness.

Understand that your value is not determined by the year your car was made. It isn't determined by whether you have the newest tablet or smartphone, a designer wardrobe or the latest hairstyle. If your friends won't like you if you don't have these things, then it is better to know now that they aren't your true friends at all. Your strengths, personality, ability to love and be loved, and uniqueness make you worthwhile. Not your possessions. And you deserve the peace of mind that comes from making good financial decisions. You deserve to sleep well at night, to smile sincerely, and to not have those worries niggling at the back of your mind all the time. You deserve it, but you need to make the right financial decisions so you can have it. No one else can do it for you, only you can do it for yourself. Chapter 8 has tools to reduce your dependence on material items for your feelings of worth or happiness.

Now let's look at sacrifice. What is it? The Oxford Dictionary defines sacrifice as "the act of giving up something valued for the sake of something else regarded as more important or worthy[5]." The Collins Dictionary states, "a surrender of something of value, as a means of gaining something more desirable or of preventing some evil[6]."

We need a combination of discipline and sacrifice to live within our means. I'm not talking about the discipline of a commander or the sacrificial attitude of a cloistered monk. We need to exercise consistent discipline with our finances. The vital step is to live within our means. By doing so, we end each month with more money, rather than running out before month's end.

Set the budget we have discussed into place, and then live by it. You may have to make sacrifices, and give up things that you like doing or having, things you cannot afford. You can put that money towards something more important that will bring peace, instead of just instant gratification. You can sleep easier at night, knowing you are taking control of your finances, and that they look much healthier.

I often see many of my clients and friends race out and buy the latest gizmo, toy, computer, smartphone, TV, or shoes. The list goes on. They feel the need to upgrade to keep up, or somehow, they will be left behind. This might be true, especially if you work in a technology field, but not to the extent that you have to camp out at the shop one or two days before a new PlayStation is released only to blow your rent money, or charge up a hefty credit card debt. People race out for that new movie or other bit of home entertainment, and pay full price–just so they can say they were among the first to get it. This is crazy! What happens to technology and entertainment products within six months of release? Their prices drop.

Another example of frivolous, impulsive spending comes from cars and houses. So often, people purchase the newest car to "enhance" their personal image. Or, they buy a house beyond their means to show off or to keep up with their friends and family. Sometimes, they do it to impress someone they don't even like.

It sounds crazy and insane when we read about it in print, doesn't it? Yet, millions do this every month. Maybe you have been amongst this crowd, at one point or another. What gets sacrificed first? Peace of mind, because the purchase often is not affordable. We really need to exercise some critical thinking here: do we really need to live in that area? Do we really need a house with three spare bedrooms? Do we really need a new car with a petrol-guzzling engine? Do we really need these things that cost more than we have to spend?

Many in my generation, and the younger generation, seem to think that when they move out of the family home, they need to maintain the same lifestyle. They feel the need to be where their parents are financially, right now, not considering where their parents started out. They forget (or haven't been told about) the decades of hard work that put their parents in a financially stable position. The parents have slowly built up to their place, yet their children want it straightaway. They will do whatever it takes, even if it means giving up peace of mind and sleep while stressing over the pressure they have created by buying big.

When my wife and I moved out, we started with a small flat. I was asked by many people, "What are you doing there? Times have changed; you don't have to live like that these days! Go get a better place." In some ways, they were right, but I had a goal to save as much as I could as fast as I could. We sacrificed the bigger, nicer, and more modern place to build our mid- and long-term financial goals, of having nice things without the accompanying stress of not being able to afford them.

I like the quote by Will Smith, "Too many people are buying things they can't afford, with money that they don't have... to impress people that they don't like!" This is only too true for so many people. If you really want to get your finances in order so that you can have peace of mind, then ask yourself, "Is this what I really need or want?" Or, "Is there a better way to get this that does not contribute to sleepless nights or family disharmony?"

Dare to Go Beyond What Others Expect of You

In the movie *What a Girl Wants*, the lead character's father is running for prime minister of England. Since she grew up in the U.S. with her mother, her father never previously knew he had a daughter. Now, he's learning fast.

She arrives in England to find her father and build a relationship with him. Because of his career and the upcoming election, she is trying hard to fit into this new world so that she does not embarrass her father. She grew up with a more relaxed, fun-filled lifestyle, and now she must learn how to behave like the English upper class. After all, she is in position to meet the Queen! She tries to adhere to their social rules, their way of doing things.

She meets a boy the locals call a "half breed". One of his parents is from the right side of town, and the other from the wrong side, causing embarrassment to the family. However, the boy's grandparents think it unfair that he would miss out on life's opportunities, so they send him to the best of schools. Still, the people from the right side of town do not like him. Meanwhile, she wants to learn how to be a respected debutant. He finally decides that he will teach her the etiquette she needs to know. Still, he asks, "Why are you trying so hard to fit in, when you were born to stand out?"

What a great question. In fact, it leads to my questions as well: Why are you trying to fit into when you really want to stand out? With whom are you trying to fit in? Why?

Think of these questions in terms of finances. Are you worried about what your family will think if you succeed financially and move forward? Or about what your friends will think? Many of my clients fear that family and friends will turn on them if they succeed financially, stab them in the back, say things like "Oh, here comes the big shot", or "Oh, you really want to mingle with the commoners now."

The fears of some clients have been well founded. Their family and friends did make these sorts of statements. When they worked through it with me, my clients developed a state of mind in which these comments eventually created little to no effect. I also have worked with clients whose families couldn't be happier for them.

Dare to be different. If you implement the actions discussed so far, such as knowing what you want, setting a goal, moving through the list of Pros and Cons, budgeting and paying cash, checking receipts, tithing charitably, paying yourself 10% for saving, and finding no need to feel guilty about progressing, you have taken the dare to be different. Understand that most people will not take these steps, because they think it is too hard.

To have the financial peace you desire, step out of your comfort zone. What is your comfort zone? Identify it, recognize it, and give yourself permission to step out of it–as well as the assurance that everything will be all right. I remember a particular job in which I wanted to get ahead. Some of my colleagues started attacking me. They would say things like, "Do you think that you are too good for us? Do you think you will be better than us out here?" Inwardly, I thought, *No, but I have goals that I want to accomplish.* Which I did.

It is up to us. Sometimes, we need to step out of our comfort zones and dare to be different. While not everyone will approve, your financial goals are worth it, so don't allow the criticism of others to stop you.

Financial Myths and Thought Processes

In order to create better financial lives, we need to understand some of the prevailing myths about money, getting rich, and the like. We likely have been taught some of these untruths in one way, shape, or form, and believe them to be true. Some are damaging to financial wealth because they influence our behavior subconsciously.

A friend of mine who thinks that money is inherently evil has come by significant sums of money several times. In every instance, she quickly finds a way to give it to family and friends, or spend it. Before she knows it, she finds herself broke again. Her thought process is directly impacting her behavior.

Some of the more common myths:

- You have to work hard for money
- Money doesn't grow on trees
- Being rich is evil

- Rich people are selfish, mean and filled with every bad quality under the sun
- You can't have money and family/love/recreation/a social life and be a good person
- I don't deserve to be financially wealthy

One of the biggest myths is that there is not enough prosperity for everyone. People either state that there is not enough food, money, or land. Think of Africa, the poorest continent on Earth. It also happens to be the most agriculturally fertile. Yet, most Africans feel they lack the resources to meet their needs. It is important to note that much of the plight facing Africans is out of their control, due to despotic governments and regimes, and the way some industrialized nations are pilfering their resources through unfair trade agreements.

However, I have heard and seen many good people avoid prosperity out of a feeling of guilt of having more than those in Africa, for example. They somehow think that because there is "not enough", them having more makes others have less.

Here's one: if you only have one thousand acres of land and one million people living on it, they can only use so much of it to raise crops and herds. Right? If two million people live on that land, you now have significantly less land to raise crops and herds. Consequently, there will not be enough food for the people. This may be true–if that is all the land you have. But look around: we have a whole world, much of it uninhabited. If people cannot grow some crop for themselves, they can exchange something that others need for food. This is not a new concept; it has sustained cultures for thousands of years. The problem is not with a lack of land, but rather, the management of resources. Several groups teach those living in impoverished areas HOW to grow crops efficiently, thus overcoming the barriers to having enough food. In this sense, many Africans have benefitted tremendously in the past ten years.

Another reason why the land/space reason is a myth is because of how much food is wasted around the world. In the U.S. alone, 40% of grown or produced food is not eaten[7]–the equivalent of 20 pounds of food is being thrown out per month, per person. Worldwide in 2011, one third of the world's global food production was lost or wasted[8]. Imagine how many hungry mouths would have benefitted!

There is enough to go around. Realistically, if you are financially empowered, able to take care of yourself, saving money, and can donate to those who lack, you are helping people more than if you remain intentionally broke.

There are other myths that we have been taught by family, friends, some religious teachings, governments and others. Many clients have been raised in a strict Christian or Catholic environment, and part of their upbringing has left them with a certain fear about attaining and sustaining wealth. After doing some research of my own, I have found that it is usually because they have either misread or not understood the teachings, or their teacher has misunderstood them. Look around: many religious leaders, ministers and pastors enjoy a great deal of personal wealth while practicing the tenets of true believers: generosity, compassion, understanding, love, forgiveness, lack of judgment. They do not flaunt what they have, but use it to extend their own ability to serve others.

Years ago, a certain church projected and enforced a lot of power over government and people. The Bible was only available in Latin, so most people couldn't understand it. Religious leaders could then say whatever they wanted (even if it was very different to what the Bible taught), and people had to follow for fear of doing wrong. Sometimes, religious leaders misled people out of accident, sometimes intentionally.

One such concept was that money was evil. One of this church's recurrent ideas was that money was evil. Therefore, to sanctify yourself, your money must be given to the church. Many draw this practice from the New Testament, in Mark 10:25[9], which talks about the eye of the needle, and how it is easier for a camel to pass through the eye of the needle than it is for a rich man to enter heaven, or enter the kingdom of God. If you consider this literally, it's impossible for a camel to pass through the eye of a needle. The implied meaning? It is impossible for a rich person to go to Heaven. For centuries, good people held on to this understanding and taught it to their children, who passed it down, and so on. Many incorrect beliefs about money resulted. Even non-religious people may think money is evil.

Now let's look at the Jewish culture and history. Their understanding is very different. At the time Mark wrote his testament, about 2,000 years ago, "the eye of the needle" was a colloquial term to describe a little entrance within the city of Jerusalem's main gate. Back then, many cities were walled to protect against marauders. The gate was guarded. At night, it would be closed. The only way in or out was through "the eye of the needle". This door was small and narrow, barely big enough for one person to squeeze through. For those who have visited the Hohensalzburg castle in Salzburg, Austria (or seen *The Sound of Music,* which was filmed in Salzburg), you might have noticed the little door built into the four-foot-thick gate; this so called eye of the needle.

For the camel to make it through the "eye of the needle", all baggage had to be removed from its back. The camel then dropped to all four knees and crawled through. Not easy, but possible. Thus, in the deeper Biblical sense, getting to Heaven means you must be humble and willing to get rid of your baggage–*sins, not money.* While I do not pretend to be a Biblical scholar, this simple research gives much more sense to the passage. The loving God I had been taught about was not going to say that you could not enter the gates of Heaven just because you had money.

Another Biblical passage that many people have quoted to me is in Timothy 6:10[10]. They say to me, the Bible says "Money is the root of all evil." I looked it up with many of these people, and showed them how they were misquoting the verse. It actually states, "The *love of money* is the root of all evil". As stated earlier in this chapter, money is neutral. It is neither good nor evil. It all depends on what we do with it.

To say money is evil is to say that a hammer is evil. Money can be used to help those in need and many other good works. Look at that certain church I mentioned. They perform good works, with many billions of dollars of so-called 'evil money', in a way no other can match. The resulting shelter, food, medical attention and services certainly didn't feel evil to the people who benefitted; they probably looked at it as a Godsend! A hammer can be used to build a house to keep those you love dry and warm. At the same time, money can be used for greedy purposes and or start wars, and a hammer can be used as a weapon to kill someone. A kitchen knife can be used to create a wonderful meal, or for committing armed robbery. I could go on and on.

My point is, money serves as a tool to make exchange easier when purchasing and selling items. It is easier to hand over a little money for some flour than to bring a lamb to exchange. What if the other person does not want a lamb, and you have nothing else to exchange? Money was created to make fair exchanges easier for people.

This next belief has nothing to do with religious upbringing, but remains a big problem: "It's a dog eat dog world". While true in many cases, this is not always the case. Some of my well-to-do friends did not get to their successful station by themselves. They worked hard and poured forth a considerable effort, but they also received help. Many said to me, "It is more of a dog-*help*-dog world out there". People that help each other get ahead, and the ones that tear each other down struggle. What is social or business networking if not people helping each other? If you want to get ahead, help other people, and allow them to help you.

Another myth: "You have to work hard for your money for your entire life". While requiring effort and discipline, it does not have to be hard. I know people that work very hard for their money, and earn well. I know others that don't work hard at all and earn the same amount. It depends on what you do to earn your money, and how you invest or save once you've earned it. There are hard ways to earn money, jobs that require lots of hours of manual labor. Mining, industrial and factory work come to mind. Others move into their adult years with their love of writing, music, art, marketing, surfing or sculpting intact, and they create solid financial lives–and love every minute of the work they do. When you find a job that feeds your expertise, and pays you more for it, then you will earn more money while probably not working as hard as before. Or, better yet, it won't feel like work at all.

The other part of the equation is to follow the saying, "Making money while you sleep." Investing your saved money creates additional earnings without any effort beyond budgeting and solid research into the fund. You deserve it. You worked for the money. Now let it work for you. Talk about a reduction in stress!

Rich People are Mean/Selfish/Nasty/Lonely/Think They Are Superior to Everyone Else

People are people. There are mean poor people. There are mean rich people. There are nice poor people. There are nice rich people. We have different personalities, different ways in which we view and treat others and methods to make our way through the world. Deep down, it doesn't matter if we are rich or poor when it comes to our core character values. Money doesn't make someone rich or poor; they would be that way regardless of their financial circumstances.

If you think that all rich people are mean, consider this: if you live in the developed world, and have a roof over your head and three meals a day, clean clothing and clean water, you are already rich according to the 1.1 billion who live without clean water[11] and almost 1 billion who live without homes or are living in slums[12]. To them, having a home, food, water and clothing is the definition of rich. Most of them live on annual incomes of less than $300. Three hundred dollars!

These myths usually arise from comments well-meaning people have said and repeated throughout your childhood and developmental years. They can influence your behavior significantly. You may have a hard time saving, or may feel guilty when prospering. You may take actions (or inactions) that get you fired. You may choose unpromising career options, because that is all you feel capable of doing. Fortunately, these harmful ideas can be remedied. Once you understand and dissolve these myths, you will see that financial abundance can be either good or bad. It all depends on how you decide to approach money, and what you do once you have it.

How to Overcome Financial Myths

Once you are aware of a myth, take steps to overcome it. What is a myth but a large, fanciful story woven from a small spool of truth or fact? One technique is to write affirmations and repeat them once a day. Think of an affirmation as a new belief or truth you want to incorporate into your life, one that will replace the myth. Affirmations like "Money is a tool I can use for good. It is good for me to be financially wealthy." Or "There is enough money and I can earn ____ (put in your goal amount)". Say your affirmations each morning after you wake up.

Another technique is to write reasons in support of your desired belief. If you wish to believe that you can have money and family (at the same time), write out the reasons why being financially wealthy helps to fulfill your role as a family member. Also write out why enjoying your family and living in a loving environment helps you have financial wealth. For example, your love for your family can drive you to perform to your best at work, to provide above and beyond. If you can write 200 reasons for each, the belief will become ingrained into your thought processes. If you want to believe that money is good, write out 200 reasons why. This is a difficult exercise if you have never thought that way, but it works.

I also help clients become aware of the situations when these myths became ingrained into their psychology. We work at dissolving the emotional and mental energy within those past situations and thought processes.

I Don't Deserve It

I will close this chapter with the worst and most stress-producing financial myth of all: "I don't deserve to be wealthy. I don't deserve to be successful. I don't deserve to (fill in the blank)." This belief arises from past guilt, a major traumatic event, or a certain upbringing.

One lady I know feels considerable guilt about mistakes she has made. When she was a young child, she ran near a road to greet her brother on the other side. He thought she was going to run onto the road, so he ran across to stop her. A speeding car hit him. His leg was broken so badly that it wrapped around his neck. His tongue was hanging on by a thread. While standing in the doorway of her home, watching emergency crews working hard to save her brother, and feeling immense fear, her mother told her "This is all your fault." Thankfully, her brother survived and recovered, but she still feels guilty for his tremendous pain and the family trauma that ensued.

She is capable of so much financial, emotional and physical goodness for herself, but often chooses the worse of two options that present themselves at any given decision-making moment. She has entered into and endured abusive relationships. She does not manage her money well, and often borrows from others to make ends meet. When she does have surplus, she spends or gives it away, instead of holding onto it for her future unexpected bills. Subconsciously, she chooses what she feels she deserves. If she learns to love herself, that she is worthy of good things, and stops blaming herself for the past, she will have a much more enjoyable life.

Guilt and self-blame can influence you in one area of life, such as finances or relationships. Or it can influence many areas at once. Either way, you are guaranteed a life of terrible stress if you walk down this path. Don't you want to rise above such a difficult road? Of course you do.

Chapter 8: Moving Into Self-Love

Lynne and Tim Martin faced an interesting dilemma. They sat in their comfortable Central California home, arguing over how to spend their retirement years. Lynne, a 69-year-old former public relations executive, and Tim, a 65-year-old former owner of a manufacturing facility, felt and acted more like teenagers with gray hair than retirees. They loved life, thoroughly enjoyed each other's company, and had adventures in which one relied upon the other for everything from emotional support to finding the next crazy experience. The last thing they wanted, or believed they deserved, was to sit in their house, look at the clock, and while away their twilight years while confining themselves to a few short trips and an endless string of doctor's appointments. That was not how they wanted to celebrate their decades-old love, one that brought them together later in life. They loved themselves and each other too much.

They make movies about love stories like Lynne's and Tim's. Maybe that will happen to this couple, since a book based on their love and travels will be released worldwide in 2014. Lynne and Tim wanted to let their wild, crazy spirits run free. Why not? They had been lovers in the late 1960s, only to create separate lives with separate partners. After a torrid romance, Lynne felt Tim's free-spirited, Bohemian songwriting lifestyle would not work for her more pragmatic, career-oriented sensibilities. While getting married to others and moving on, they never lost that special beat of the heart for each other.

Fast forward to 2003: Lynne's husband, Guy, suffered from late-stage Alzheimer's disease. Tim's marriage, which produced three beautiful daughters, now in their 30s and early 40s, had ended. On a whim, he drove four hours north from Los Angeles to the Central Coast, and made a surprise visit to Lynne and Guy. Remember that special beat of the heart? Sure enough, it kicked up again. Given the situation in Lynne's life, these two people of highest integrity bonded by pouring love into Guy during his "long sunset," as late U.S. President Ronald Reagan described his Alzheimer's. With Tim's friendship and encouragement, Lynne's enormous stress level reduced so completely that she was able to shift her self-love from protecting her heart to pouring it into Guy. She transformed her stress into love. This went on for three years, until Guy passed away.

In 2008, Lynne and Tim were married. So it was then, that they arrived at that critical point: live out their retirement in one house, worrying about medical issues and bank accounts and growing old? Or, as Lynne recalls, "Do we do something that will make our friends and families think we have gone off the hook, totally crazy?"

They felt so sure of themselves, so in love with each other and life itself, that they chose the latter. They spent a year planning their "great escape," sold their house and most of their possessions, let their families know their intentions – "There were plenty of tears and rolling of eyes," Lynne says – and they hit the road. They figured that it would cost less to live in places around the world, than to incur living expenses, medical bills, and the stress of staying alive without working in ultra-expensive California. Not to mention the stress of two big personalities with high energy and plenty of collective ADHD trying to navigate around each other with nothing but the next meal in their plans.

For the past three years, they have lived in twenty different cities and locales, staying for one to three months at a time, renting apartments in places such as San Miguel de Allende and Buenos Aires, beach houses near Lisbon and Cornwall, villas in Tuscany and Marrakech, a room within a 300-year-old Georgian manor in Ireland, and flats in London, Istanbul and along the Seine in their favorite destination, Paris. They have grown happier and more full of life, if that's even possible, despite dealing with countless stressors like rescheduling cruises, dealing with rental agencies, broken-down rental cars, errant GPS devices, the horrors of driving in southern Italy, eating unsettling food, misplacing keys, taking overnight flights to Istanbul without their pickup driver turning up, losing credit cards, fighting bad weather, failing to get Internet connections when planning next destinations, and cultural impasses that left them wondering why they took on lives better spent by young adults trying to find themselves overseas.

The Martins' journey likely will not end until one or the other becomes infirmed, something they seem to be pushing further into the future. South America, Australia, New Zealand and south Asian countries are in line for the next couple of years. Both feel younger than they have in two decades. Their sense of courage in jumping into the next fire – the next new place, the next new set of local customs and cultural mores, the next language – has drawn praise from many thousands of people who follow their adventures on Lynne's blog. It has also earned Lynne a major book contract – at age 72.

Most of all, the necessity of relying upon each other in foreign lands, again and again, has brought a strength in their relationship that, Tim says, "Keeps us as madly in love as when we were young lovers, only a lot deeper and seasoned by what I hope is greater wisdom."

Lynne and Tim sound like young lovers when they talk about each other. Isn't that wonderful? In their story resides a grand example of what happens when you cultivate a high level of self-esteem and self-love, and a fair bit of courage. Lynne could have easily shrunk into quiet widowhood. Tim could have faced his later life with soul-crushing loneliness, and its attendant health-threatening stress, when his marriage ended in his early 60s.

Instead, this couple turned possible stressful futures into a fabulous outcome that has its moments–and arguments–but thrives on a foundation that mitigates stress, promotes health and vitality, and sees the silver lining in every situation. Their foundation is self-esteem and self-love, the greatest of stress-reducing inner qualities and the primary subtheme of this book.

The Self-Opinion–Stress Relationship

In my years of consulting, I have arrived at what I believe to be the "genesis" cause of much inner stress and unease, if you will, the one factor that pulsates through everything else: *a lot of stress results from a lack of self-esteem and self-love.* A lot of stress comes from the effects of guilt and a low opinion of yourself, because the negative effects of low self-opinion spread into other areas of our lives like wildfire.

This happens in two ways. Firstly, when we do not feel strong and confident about ourselves, outside circumstances or events seep in more readily. Sometimes, they become downright toxic. Holes are poked into our self-esteem and psyche, and aggravate or frustrate us. Stress frequently follows. Of course, it is not the only source, but when our self-opinion and self-confidence are low, that inner frustration is automatically and unknowingly projected outwards. We get frustrated with outer circumstances and other people more easily. As a result our overall stress levels are higher, and our opinion on life is less than ideal. Life's joys pass us by more easily, and our relationships suffer.

Secondly, when self-opinion and self-love are low, we allow or even accept stressful circumstances into our lives. I see so many people accepting less than what they deserve when their self-esteem falls (or is already low) and their ability to deal with stress is reduced. It is like starting from the top of the stairs, taking a few steps down, and then thinking you're as high up the staircase as you'll ever go again. Then, when the next stressful

event hits and shakes you up, you slide down three more steps–
and think you can go no higher.

So many people have experienced this slide–many after
achieving early success and opportunity in their lives. The global
financial crisis and ensuing recession of 2008-2012 sent countless
millions of people into lifestyles beneath what they'd known
before. Question is, how did they handle it? For those who
crumble under stress, and continue to slide down that staircase,
their new life is fueled by a reduced self-opinion and complicated
by more stress. Their dreams seem a universe away. How can
they love themselves when their life hopes have been crushed?
When the very thing they base their feelings of self-worth on
(material success) has vanished?

But here's the thing: while millions worldwide can use the
global financial crisis as a strong excuse for their downslide,
millions of others were already down this rabbit hole because
they held a low self-opinion in general. Often, for their entire
lives. It is this group that most needs an approach to deal with
stress and see the love and value of life.

People in this group often feel that the situations they live
with are normal, and just reflect what life is like. Or, they may
believe that the situations they endure are all that is possible for
them. They want something better for themselves, and wonder
why they constantly end up with the raw end of the deal when
others have it so easy. Despite the fact that they really are
incredibly amazing in their own way, low self-opinion has a toxic
effect on their lives.

These lives often play out in the following ways: Abusive
relationships. Imbalanced or dysfunctional relationships.
Situations where they are taken for granted. Low paying jobs
with no goal of progression. Mistreatment at work. Not giving to
themselves financially, by not saving. Going out of their way to
help others at incredible expense to themselves. Walking through
life with shoulders slumped, head down, and "poor me" written

between the lines on their foreheads and the bags beneath their eyes. Letting others talk down to them in a condescending, character-crushing way. Never voicing their opinions–or, when they do, they tend to make self-deprecating statements like, "I know my opinion doesn't really matter, but ..."

If you ask them if they deserve better, they usually reply that of course they do. But if you dig deeply, you find that deep down, they feel they are getting all that they deserve. When dealing with those who once sat atop their careers, marriages, and stature in society or the world, we try to remind them nicely of *what* got them into those positions–in nearly all cases, strong self-esteem and self-love, and the confidence that ensues. They often reply, "Well, that was before the world kicked me down, and kicked me, and kicked me... I just can't take it anymore." And, sadly, they truly believe they cannot. Their self-opinion has eroded to next to nothing. For those who never possessed a strong self-opinion in the first place, the task to build self-love and self-confidence becomes even more important.

Not every instance of abuse or mistreatment is a direct result of low self-esteem. However, in most instances it does play a large role. When you have a healthy respect for yourself, you are not vulnerable to or romantically attracted to abusive personalities. When mistreatment begins to occur, you are able to see the signs when they first appear, instead of well down the road when it is too late. If you don't have the knowledge you need to solve the situation immediately, you can quickly attain it. This is why improving self opinion is so helpful in breaking patterns of abuse or continual mistreatment.

The good thing is, having a low self-opinion is not permanent. It can be changed. Your opinion and love for yourself can be improved, and when you do, your happiness improves too. You become empowered in your personal circumstances, and have more power to resolve stressful circumstances–and prevent them in the first place.

Remember the story of Rebecca from Chapter 2? She is a prime example of this. Due to molestation and the terrible things said to her as a child, her self-loathing, and lack of self-love, were extreme. However, today she is a confident woman. She holds a great degree of self-respect and self-love. Circumstances have occurred where others have begun to encroach upon her newly set boundaries, but she has not allowed others to bully or overpower her. Rebecca has been able to prevent the stress that comes from being taken for granted, because of her increased self-love.

Self-Sabotage

Now let's look closer at where true self-love, self-esteem and self-opinion go awry–and open the floodgates for stress to do its corrosive work. On a conscious level, you might want a nice house, a good relationship, or a job where you are paid fairly and which offers further skills training or advancement opportunities. You may even put a lot of effort into achieving goals, connecting your sense of purpose to the project, or the position. This is good. Everything that is produced with quality and excellence requires good effort. You must put forth the energy to achieve anything positive in your life.

At the same time, however, your true inner opinion of yourself will influence your actions. If we have a low self-opinion, our habits and actions can sabotage our efforts at what we want– a happy relationship, good relations with our children, a fulfilling career, and any number of other good, worthwhile outcomes. This is the *why*–why low self-opinion causes a lot of stress.

The habits and thoughts you gained in childhood, reinforced in adolescence and carried into your adult life will also impact the result. If you threw temper tantrums as a child or teenager, never worked out the root causes, and are hit with a stressful situation or confronted by someone you dislike, how will you react? Likely, you will lash back in some way, with a sharp comment or a physical outburst. Our unresolved childhood or adolescent traits will fly out of seemingly nowhere, reflecting low self-opinion and lack of control even though we may seem completely together and confident on the surface.

Likewise, if you deeply believe, in your heart and soul that you don't deserve a certain result, or have fears about it, you may become your own worst enemy. The story of one of my clients illustrates this perfectly. She came to me with a lot of weight issues which, when you consider her devotion to exercise, was surprising at first glance. She exercised every day. She ran in the morning or evening. She worked out in the gym several times a week. She also followed a strict diet, eating healthy, balanced dinners with an emphasis on vegetables. She ate fish often, and kept her portion sizes relatively small. No matter how hard she exercised or how much she counted calories on her nutritional diet, though, she kept putting on weight. At one point, she gained about 10 kilos (22 pounds) in three weeks – *despite* a fitness and eating regimen which would be the envy of many marathon runners, let alone everyday people trying to lose weight.

At that point, she came to me for help. We spoke about what she was doing physically to lose weight. We spoke about what attaining and maintaining a healthy weight meant to her, and why she *really* wanted it. After that, we started to talk about what it meant to her on a deeper level. We uncovered some of her fears and inner feelings about living at a consistently healthy weight, utilizing questioning techniques I learned from my core qualification and from continued study and research, which have been refined over the years.

The answers surprised both of us. When she was a young teenager, a trusted friend told her that thin, pretty girls tend to get raped. Imagine being 13 or 14, an age when saying "hello" in a certain tone can cause angst for a teenaged girl, and having one of your best friends dislodge every healthy notion you possessed about looking good. Needless to say, this made an impression deep within my client. Even though she wanted to be thin and "pretty", her body reacted at the cellular level, and did absolutely everything in its power to prevent her from being viewed as a potential rape victim – or even someone attractive. Her thyroid and metabolism slowed down. Her healthy diet and exercise habits did not counteract her hypoactive thyroid at all. In fact, the more she tried to lose weight, the more weight she put on!

We worked through her fear. I helped her see that both the statement and her perception of it were false. We tweaked her diet ever so slightly, and I also worked on her acupressure points to help stimulate her thyroid. She continued to work on losing weight, and finally began to see results. Without the severe block of "if I'm pretty, I'll get raped" stifling her thyroid and metabolism, both returned to levels consistent with people who work out regularly and eat wisely. It happened quickly, too–far more quickly than some dietary adjustments and work on acupressure points would normally provide. She lost the weight that she had rapidly gained, plus additional weight she had carried for years. She accomplished all of this without taking any pharmaceutical fat burning or weight loss products.

In this client's case, fear impacted her weight. But the cause of a negative stress-induced reaction is not always fear. Quite often, it is your opinion about what you are worth, what you deserve, and whether certain things are possible for you to attain. Such as, "Why do I work my tail off to barely make ends meet, while the guy I grew up with plays golf four days a week, and rakes in millions of dollars? Why does he have the Midas touch, and I don't?" Or, "Why do I want a loving relationship more than anyone I know, and yet, they enjoy solid longstanding relationships and I keep falling in and out of mine?"

Let's meet another client. She seemed to experience one bad relationship after another. Every guy she dated seemed great, but after dating him for a while, she would inevitably discover he was also dating someone else. Worse than that, he *wanted* to be with the other person–and was only dating her *as a fallback plan* in case it didn't work out with the person he really wanted. To make matters worse, while she dated a succession of these men (before she learned they were dating someone else), she would go above and beyond to give them the very best of herself and her life. She would pay for the dates, drive long distances to see them, and pour her heart into every conversation, activity and intimate moment. In short, she did all the work, all the giving.

When I met this lady, I would not have guessed her to be in such a predicament. I found her to be a truly great woman, the type of person whose company any balanced, sensible man with self-esteem and a respect for women would enjoy. She was honest, fair, kind, a good worker, and both capable of and well-practiced at doing almost anything for those close to her. She was great at organizing social events with her friends, and fun to be around. She didn't fly off the handle and unload with emotional outbursts or dump her baggage – even when she realized how badly these guys had really treated her. She felt she deserved and wanted a decent man who would be honest with her, take their relationship seriously, deal with any disagreements or issues upfront, and treat her with respect.

However, when we moved to her inner issues, I found an entirely different atmosphere – and a lot of reasons why she felt she didn't deserve a man capable of sharing a long relationship, or a life-long relationship: i.e., events from her past that she felt guilty about and negative things people had said about her as a child – things she had believed. All those things had chipped away at her self-respect to the point that she was attracted to men that treated her in a way that confirmed her inner thoughts.

Through the processes described in this book, her life has turned around. She is happy with herself, and has let go of her guilt. She also doesn't fall for selfish men any more. In fact, she has found an honest, fair, kind-hearted, devoted and overall loving man, and they are happily married. They work through their challenges together, and he is the type of man many women dream of.

Saboteurs of Self-Love

Out of the variety of factors which corrode our self-opinion, perhaps none is more corrosive than guilt. Guilt can be defined as self-directed anger. It comes from the perception that we have made a mistake or were somehow not good enough. I am not talking about the appropriate sorrow one feels after causing another pain–the sorrow that prompts us to remedy a situation, and then is alleviated once we do. The guilt I am referring to is carried on well after the event is corrected, and can range from self-blame to outright self-disgust.

Most of us experience guilt at one time or another. Usually this is over past events where we see that we have caused another pain. On the outside, we shrug it off, and justify to ourselves that it is not a big deal and that they will get over it, or that they deserved it anyway. On the inside however, it eats at us. Most of the time, we are completely unaware that this guilt is still there, but every now and then, an event happens, or someone says something, and we are reminded of the guilt that we feel as it temporarily comes to our recollection.

This guilt can also come from situations where we felt we weren't good enough. Where we weren't quite "up to scratch". Perhaps our perceived inadequacy has caused problems in our lives–"If only I had been more confident in that interview, I would have gotten that job" or "If only I had spoken up, then I could have helped her get out of that abusive situation" or even "If only I had worked harder in school, I could have had a better career" These past 'mistakes' can erode our self-respect each time we think about them.

Learned Self Blame

Another major source of lowered self-opinion is learned self-blame. This is where, as a conditioned response, we blame ourselves for situations (even those not really under our control).

Several of my clients have overcome this habit. One, for example, would apologize when a minor hiccup occurred, such as another person being late. Or when a movie was cancelled, that a group of people had planned to see, one of my clients would apologize for the situation. It sounds silly, but she had learned to assume responsibility *and blame* for situations that had nothing to do with her.

While the above situations seem insignificant, they served as an indicator of her outlook on life, which extended to much more significant events. If someone was exercising power over her, and she tried to set boundaries, causing the offender to become aggressive, she would blame herself for the aggressor's reaction. She would literally take blame for another person's emotional response. In fact for any conflict situation she was a part of, she would automatically blame herself. In fact, she would automatically assume blame for any conflict situation involving her, regardless of how big or small her role was in the situation. On the one hand, she felt angry at the other person, and felt it was all the other person's fault. But on the other hand, she felt extremely guilty for her role in the situation, even if she was not out of line.

This pattern of self-blame can stem from parents unknowingly – or even worse, knowingly - shaming their children. To a child, who is like a sponge in its formative years, many less-than-best parenting behaviors actually teach guilt and blame. Excessively pointing out a child's mistakes, as a form of discipline, accomplishes this. Yes, accountability needs to be learned, but using a loud or overly firm voice while stating the mistakes the child has made, only teaches them to be externally defensive and to internally assume blame.

Likewise, parents getting angry over mistakes causes problems. Think about how big and loud you feel when you are mad. To a child, who is physically smaller, this effect is amplified. The result? Children feel that they are not good enough, or they are deficient as a person, when they make a mistake. Not that the behavior isn't good enough; it's that they feel *they* aren't good enough. Even tones of voice that express disappointment, used repetitively, can enforce this message. On the outside children appear to grow immune, even increasingly rebellious, but the effects come out in full force in adult life. These seemingly harmless parenting behaviors can cause harmful adult stress.

Of course, I do not condone letting children run wild and withholding discipline all together. There are approaches to parenting that involve calm and effective discipline without guilt and shame. I personally have found that my children become more cooperative, happier, and *more responsible* for their actions when my wife and I put effort into these methods. No one is perfect and parental mistakes happen, despite the best efforts. In these times it is best to not exercise your own self-blame, but to carry on and learn from your mistake. If your overall parenting approach is calm yet effective, occasional accidental shame messages have a much smaller impact on a child's feelings of self-worth.

Learned self-blame is probably most powerful when it originates in traumatic events or abuse. To tell a child "this is all your fault" after a major accident is to pass down a potential life sentence of guilt. The lady whose story is found at the end of Chapter 7 is a perfect example of this. Young children can also blame themselves for their parents' divorce, an event which is very traumatic in their eyes.

Abusers often deliberately use blame as a tool to keep their victims from speaking out. Statements like "This is all your fault", "No one will believe you if you tell them" or "You will get in trouble if you tell" are just the beginning of the guilt complexes that come from molestation and abuse. Thankfully, all of my clients have been able to overcome (or are in the process of overcoming) powerfully learned self-blame, even when it has stemmed from intense childhood situations.

How We Measure Our Worth

Another very common factor which corrodes our self-opinion is the society wide trend of comparing our results with the success of others, particularly when our results are less impressive than those around us. Sometimes, the things we compare are unattainable illusions, yet we still compare ourselves to them. For example, there is no point trying to measure up to "Photoshopped" or airbrushed images of celebrities, yet millions of us do it! Or we compare our current circumstances to outcomes which are a result of long term success. Despite our own strengths, we feel insecure and not quite good enough. Perhaps the most common areas people compare themselves in are physical appearance (weight, figure, muscle tone, facial features) and material success (cars, houses, bank account sizes, job titles). This all comes at a cost of lowered self-esteem. If we base our feelings of self-worth on success in these areas (another society-wide trend), then our self-opinion takes an even bigger blow.

I had a conversation with a mentor who helps people deal with and overcome stress. He was telling me of a client, an entrant in a top beauty pageant. She saw my mentor because she thought that there was something wrong with her breasts. My mentor said that, in his mind, there was nothing wrong. When he asked more questions, he found out what she was comparing herself to. Then he helped her through her issue, and she grew to be happy with herself.

This example illustrates an important point. Here was a truly beautiful young lady with the world at her fingertips and even *she* compared herself to some ideal!

When something happens to diminish our success, such as ageing, not getting exercise time, or financial challenges (as many experienced during the recent recession), the problem escalates. For example, a man works 30 years to provide for his family, saves a couple hundred thousand dollars–and it vanishes in the snap of his fingers due to a backroom decision made by the multinational conglomerate running the corporation for which he works. And just what was the fateful decision that made this hard earned money disappear? The board decided to cover their losses with employees' 401(k) and other pension funds.

Let's assume this man then finds out his home value is underwater–he owes more on the mortgage than the house is worth. Suddenly, at age 55, everything he's worked for is gone. Since he measured his self-worth by his work, and his meticulous plan for retirement, he's ruined emotionally.

If our entire notion of self-worth and purpose is based on success in one of these areas, and that area suffers, our self-opinion can topple faster than a toddler's tower of blocks. This explains the historical high suicide rates during a recession–the stress of financial loss and blow to one's self-opinion can seem too much to deal with. In my experience, it also contributes to the depression that sufferers of chronic illness feel when they are suddenly unable to fulfill family responsibilities or their perceived purpose in life.

Improving Self-Opinion and Self-Love

When I talk to clients about their self-opinion, I usually initially receive a firm or even defensive response: "I don't suffer from a lack of self-esteem. I know I love myself." They are right–*to the extent they recognize self-esteem or self-love.* This is not necessarily the same as having low self-esteem. You probably don't think that you have low self-esteem. You probably feel that you have the normal amount of self-esteem.

At the same time, though, how highly do you really value yourself? Do you feel like you can be the very best at what you do? Are you doing your best every day, because you have to in order to please others? Or because you *want* to, to please yourself? Do you look around and say, "I am so entirely in love with my spouse that I feel the love from everyone and everything around me"? Or, "I take care of myself because I want to be at my best to live to my fullest potential"? Or, the *carpe diem* approach: "Today, I am going to seize every moment because I deserve the best, and everyone deserves the best I have to give–no matter what challenges or obstacles happen along the way"? Or the simplest test of all: is it easy for you to think of 10 good things about yourself, right now, in the next 30 seconds?

Our knee-jerk reaction is to automatically say a resounding "Yes" to all of these questions. Of course! Who *doesn't* want to operate at their best, love deeply or make the most out of life?

However, if we are being honest with ourselves, these questions are a little more difficult to answer. Most of us do not truly hold ourselves in high esteem or love ourselves in the way we really deserve. Our competitive natures and an even more competitive society and business climate suggest that self-esteem results from believing "I'm better than them", "My kids are the best in the school at everything", or "Nobody's taking the contract from me today". This is not self-esteem, but comparative actions built on pride, a totally different story.

Self-esteem measures itself in a healthy respect for yourself. You don't need to tell anyone how much you love, how accomplished you are, or how warmly others regard you during a dinner party, school function or night out with friends. When you hold high self-esteem, people often sense it. Your optimism toward life and your positive energy make it very clear. You have setbacks, negatives and challenges in life, but you put in the effort to overcome them. Nothing can hold you back. You even look for what the challenge can teach you, how you can learn from it. You deal with twists and turns by seeking out the heart of any stressor–with a resolution to overcome it. Or at least a positive attitude. No matter what the situation, or predicament, you can find the confidence, resolution or gentle touch that is required to de-stress it. Or, if you don't have the answers, you confidently turn to someone who does, and ask the right questions.

People gravitate to you. Your positive energy and sense of self-love and self-esteem is a strong attractor. Many will want to socialize with you and spend time within your positive energy. Even those who may not like you will come to hold respect for you, even if they try to tear you down first. People will admire you, feel better for knowing you, and even turn to you for insight or advice on matters in which your experience can help them. Outside opinions won't matter as much to you, because you have learned how to deal with criticism and find the positive aspects of it. Your self-worth is not dependent on others. Through all of this, you do not feel the need to boast about your life, or accomplishments. *That* is healthy respect for self. *That* is high self-esteem. That is the goal of the following exercises.

How to Improve Self-Love

To quickly improve self-opinion, I help clients to recognize the events from their past where they carry guilt, and resolve the self-blame associated with it. This enables them to make the big changes that have been spoken about in this chapter quite quickly.

I also give the following exercises as reinforcement to the mental shifts made in consultations. When used alone, these activities will help to gradually improve self-opinion. At first the improvement may seem small, but over time the impact adds up. Many clients have reported months down the track that they are now so much happier and far less stressed than before they began these techniques.

Turning Perception Around

A common effect of stress is to see only the bad in situations, to see what is frustrating us. However, this only adds to the stress that we feel. When we are in this frame of mind, we don't notice many of the great things around us. We miss out on some of the joys life has to offer us. The purpose of this first exercise is to turn that around, to start noticing those good things and feel the happiness and gratitude that comes from noticing them.

Activity 1: Each day, write out ten things you are grateful for. It may be events from that day, or people or circumstances you are glad to have in your life. They need to be different things each day. If this is a difficult exercise for you, it indicates that your conscious focus is on the negative, the stressful, and you really need to do this activity!

The purpose of the second and third exercises is to increase the amount of good things you see in yourself. This directly serves to increase feelings of self-worth and shift the focus away from your perceived faults, to your strengths. Again, the effects are gradual, but my clients have noticed significant changes in happiness and stress levels through these activities. These exercises have been instrumental in breaking through lifetime patterns of self-blame and moving on to accept better circumstances and greater joy and happiness.

Activity 2: Each day, write out ten good things about yourself. They can be good things that you did that day, or good character points in general. Write different things every day. Once again, if this is a difficult exercise, it indicates your conscious awareness is based on your downfalls, and you need to do this exercise!

Activity 3: Think of a statement that describes how you want to think about yourself. You can point out your character strengths or skills, such as "I am confident, caring, and friendly. I have good work ethic and am innovative" or "I am a worthwhile person. I contribute to the world in ways that only I can." Form a statement, and repeat it to yourself at least three times each day.

An easy way to remember to do activities one, two and three is to incorporate them into your routine. You can do these activities while you are driving, doing housework, waiting on the elevator, or in the checkout line. Any time that you don't need to put mental effort into another task is a great opportunity to improve your self-opinion through these activities.

Through the final exercise, we are going to work on dissolving that residual guilt that can linger due to past events. If you have guilt over an event where you caused another person pain (aside from calmly setting your own boundaries), do what you can to remedy the situation, to make amends. This often alleviates guilt and brings peace. However, sometimes guilt can still remain, especially over events from years ago where it may not be possible to make amends now, or if you really think you had a negative impact on someone's life.

In these situations, you can resolve guilt by seeing how your mistake benefitted the other person. Remember the positive side of stressful situations? Just as you have learnt and grown from your stressful experiences, the stress you have caused others has given them an opportunity to learn and grow. This doesn't justify deliberately causing others stress for the sake of giving them learning experiences, but it does help to shift your mind away from self-condemnation over past events. Start by thinking of at least ten ways your action benefitted the other person, and continue thinking of benefits until you feel at peace about the situation. For example, did they learn resilience? Did they become independent? Did they learn to trust their instinct above yours?

And what is the positive impact of those things in their life? Has it helped them to make their own decisions? To excel professionally? It is amazing how the mistakes of one person can become the seeds of strength of character and greatness in another. For example, one of my clients felt significant guilt about how unkind she was to her sister as a teenager. Even after apologizing years later, she still felt guilty to the point that it was impacting her life. However through doing this exercise she realized that her unkindness actually helped her sister to become the independent and resilient person she is today. Her sister is now quite successful professionally, exceling in management roles due to her independence and resilience during stressful circumstances.

A lot of us aim for perfection, which is a great goal. But we expect ourselves to be perfect today, and this can exacerbate our guilt when we make mistakes, by adding the self-disappointment of not meeting that expectation (perfection). But perfection is a process! If we were meant to be instantly perfect, we would have been born instantly perfect. But how did we start out life? Falling down, landing on our faces, crying as toddlers, and perhaps even hitting other children. Then hopefully we learned to control our actions, communicate our needs without crying, and get along with others. Likewise, we are still learning and growing today. Life is a learning process, and you are still learning. If you made a mistake in the past, give yourself the same grace, the same benefit of the doubt, that you would your best friend if they made a mistake. You deserve it.

Chapter 9: Conquering Fear & Stress

One day, friends talk you into doing something you never imagined – jumping off a 10-meter cliff into a lake. You swim well, and you enjoyed diving off the 3-meter board during your teenage years, but this is a different story. Well, two *more* stories, if you take the average height of a high-rise floor. However, with a spot of courage and a desire to try new experiences, you choose to join them.

Everything feels great about the day and the jump–until you climb the trail that leads to the cliff. As you walk, worst-case scenario questions pop into your head: what if I jump into a shallow spot? What if I slip and don't launch myself away from the rocky face? What if I look down while in mid-air and do a belly flop? What if I hit my head on something underwater? What if my foot gets jammed in a rock on the bottom and I can't swim back up? What if…

By the time you reach the top of the cliff, your mind has run more movies of what can go wrong than a film festival. Then you take your first look over the cliff – and your body freezes. Your heartbeat speeds into hummingbird range. Cold sweat beads on your forehead, even though it's 30º C (86º F) outside. Your mind screams out, *I'm going to get hurt! I'm going to become paralyzed! I'm going to die!*

You approach the cliff again, start to jump–and stop. You try again–and stop again. The fear begins to overwhelm you, tightening everything from your muscles to thought processes. You can't remember ever feeling this much physical stress. Mentally, could it possibly be more stressful? All of this, over a cliff jump? You want to laugh yourself off the planet.

Finally, after more prodding by your friends, you close your eyes… and jump. Two seconds later, you hit the water, pencil straight, bob back to the surface, and swim to shore. The rush of wind… the speed of descent… the thrill of being airborne… the pleasing shock of hitting cool water… what a blast! You scramble up the cliff trail and jump again – and again – and again. Each time feels better than before. Soon, you're kicking your legs out, hooting and hollering as you leap, and sprinting off the cliff like an Olympic long jumper. Now you're thinking, "Why on Earth was I so scared?"

How many times have we asked ourselves that question? How many times have we worked ourselves into a frenzy, or brought ourselves to the point of paranoia and sheer fright, before taking that next step and realizing we had nothing to worry about? We have many things to fear in life – or so we think. Life issues present far more serious concerns than jumping off a 10-meter cliff, that's for sure. We fear losing our own or our children's safety, finances, old secrets being revealed, losing our spouses or loved ones, losing our jobs… even waking up and having to face the next day. The list goes on. Unless we are beyond fear itself, everyone has a list of some size. With each of those experiences, we shave off a bit of ourselves. That's because of the intense stress generated, along with flight-or-fight hormones (cortisol and adrenaline) and the impact they make on our minds and bodies.

A great deal of stress comes from fear. There are two major ways fear presents itself in our lives: through the comfort zones we establish, and through the stressful events we experience. Both can involve deep-rooted fears. Take the cliff jumper. His comfort zone for jumping into water, locked in during his teenaged years, stopped at three meters. By climbing to 10 meters, he was well out of his zone. The act of climbing the trail, thinking about the jump, and then facing its potentially negative consequences – real and imagined – took his fear to the edge of panic. In his case, fear manifested in both ways.

In both situations, we can overcome our fear and move on. Most of it can be resolved by asking yourself a basic question: "Why does this bother me?" This helps you identify the fear. You can then dissolve some of the tension by thinking objectively and rationally about an approach for dealing with the situation. If fear shows us anything, it would be how potentially irrational and illogical our minds can be when wild mental scenarios, cortisol and adrenaline take over.

In my work, I help clients find connections in their lives to see where the problem has happened before. I also help them overcome the related fear and pain they felt as children, or in a past relationship or situation. This is very helpful at stopping the fear response from triggering in current situations. When an element of fear continues to happen, clients can mentally override it and reassure themselves. We can then work toward the state of well-being in which that fear response doesn't happen at all.

Comfort zone fears sometimes relate to childhood or past traumas, but not always. They can also be created and locked in because of the conditions surrounding our developmental years or through our adult life experiences. Many people view their comfort zone as the place from which to conduct their entire lives, but truth is, great achievers and people who overcome fear view comfort zones merely as harbors. They dock themselves, make the needed adjustments, take on a load of courage, and head back to the wide open world stronger than ever.

One of my clients wanted to be financially wealthy. However, he'd had past negative business experiences. He ran a very successful company before his business partner ran off with the cash. He was held legally liable, and personally lost everything due to the collapse of the business. For years, he struggled financially, but wanted to be successful again. He worked throughout, but kept getting jobs where he wasn't paid well. When we worked through it, he realized he now had a smaller comfort zone, where he felt comfortable on lower incomes. He had associated wealth with the risk of feeling the pain again that he and his family suffered when he lost the business. He had to overcome his fear of failure. Eventually, he found work in a well paying job, where he is paid honestly and fairly. He is now doing well financially.

Stressful Events

Fear is the perception that we will incur more pain than pleasure in a particular situation. We assume that we will have a negative experience. That alone creates stress. A situation can remind us of a past stressful experience, where we think we experienced more pain than pleasure. This draws us back into that same fear response we endured during past stressful events. We may also fear it happening again, or receiving the same negative result. The result: the volcano effect. Our fear builds until finally, it blows – and spews molten emotions on our lives and the lives of those around us.

Tama was a client of mine who suffered from an unresolvable hamstring and shoulder injury which wouldn't heal. He had been injured for over a year and a half. Before being hurt, he was a professional rugby player, the star of his team, and a likely candidate to advance to international competition. He had already received a lot of medical and physiotherapeutic attention to help him recover, but to no avail. He wanted to be back on the field and live up to everyone's expectations that were put on him, (particularly his uncle's).

When we discussed his situation, Tama said that he didn't think he would be good enough to go international once he fully recovered. Everyone else thought he was good enough, and everyone else could see it, but Tama couldn't. Deep down, he feared *becoming* an international player, and then letting everyone down once he was there. He also feared that once he lived up to these expectations, even higher expectations might follow.

We worked through his fear. I helped him come to terms with it, and then overcome it. He rose above his fear of letting others down, as well as pleasing them instead of himself. He never wanted to progress as far as he did; originally, he wanted to play recreationally. We made physical corrections and engaged in activities to help his muscles heal, contract and relax properly. These helped hold his joints in place properly.

After four weeks, Tama had overcome his fears. He wanted to go back to rugby on his own terms. He felt that, if he was selected for the next level, he would be able to choose for himself whether or not to go, instead of doing it so he wouldn't let others down. At the same time, he also enjoyed a major physical recovery. He felt no pain, his hamstring recovered, and he had full range of motion and strength in his shoulder. His team physiotherapist cleared him to play.

Our fears can run (and ruin) our lives. They are often the reason why we react badly to situations. The event that causes fear or stresses you may not be stressful for someone else, who hasn't faced the same past experiences that formed the fears or created the baggage.

Another example comes from a woman who visited me after enduring countless arguments with her husband. She was angry and upset because he left the house without telling her where he was going, and she reacted angrily with yelling and anger. Her fear response kicked in. Deep down, her husband's decisions to leave reminded her of feelings of abandonment as a child. Back then, her father would come home late, and her mother would not know where he was. She would react angrily when he returned. Before he returned, several unanswered questions brought uncertainty into the home: Where was he? What was he doing? Who was he doing it with? This uncertainty was amplified by her mother's accompanying irritability.

Now my client felt the same uncertainty as her mother. She wanted her husband to always tell her of his whereabouts so she felt more secure. As a result, she reacted angrily to keep him from leaving without telling her his whereabouts. However, her angry reaction did not solve the problem; it only exacerbated it. Her husband would not listen to her needs, not because he didn't care, but because *she was not communicating them adequately.*

When she realized how their current situation related to the pain she felt as a child, she calmed down. She learned more effective ways of communicating, and forged an agreement with her husband. He still occasionally leaves without telling her where he is going, but she reminds herself everything is OK and mentally overrides her old feelings of fear and neglect.

Losing Control

Before we can learn to master our fears and stresses, we need to understand what happens when they master us. When we allow our fears to rule us, we worry about what someone else might think, or what might happen if we fail. Consequently, we limit our ability to do the job or to take the right action. Worse, we grind our teeth and shake over the possibility that we *might* fail… and let that fear take control of us. Our stress level rises, and that feeling of "analysis paralysis" and tunnel vision stress takes hold. Consequently, we spend more and more time thinking about why we are not doing it. Think of salesmen on a cold streak, knowing they have to make cold calls to open up their pipeline of leads again – yet hating the thought of talking to an unfamiliar voice who could easily tell them to get lost. How many hits can an ego take? So they spend the day rearranging piles of paper on their desks, and tormenting themselves over a future experience whose outcome *they cannot possibly know.*

This illustrates an outcome we all want to avoid. When a situation gets bad enough, and our fear builds long enough, we start to spiral. Spiraling often starts slowly, and we don't even know it is happening at first. We try to deal with what has happened, or perhaps run from what is happening. We spin more quickly. Before we know it, we feel out of control.

Heated arguments between partners, or co-workers, offer classic examples of situations that spiral out of control. Who would think that a misheard remark, a single unsavory comment, or a misread facial expression, would lead to a blowout that tears up both people? Under normal circumstances, an explanation, apology and quick chat would remedy the situation. When stress and fear grip one or both parties, misunderstandings arise. Things are said. It spirals into a loud shouting match, a real mess.

One symptom of spiraling is the magnification of our problems. We feel that our problem is so real and massive that we have no control over it. We see it as more than the sum of its parts. We believe the problem exceeds our ability to deal with it. It weighs down on us until we end up with a feeling of hopelessness. No matter what we do, we cannot solve the problem, and we're going to be stuck in this position. Ever feel that way? We all have.

However, this perception is not the actual case. When you look at your life, you will see that you have picked yourself up and emerged from tough situations over and over again. In the vast majority of cases, you emerged stronger and wiser, with less to fear and more to achieve. When we exaggerate our problems, we cloud our judgment. We negatively reinforce a perceived inability to prevail, because it becomes more difficult to make the best decision. We actually believe our exaggerations to be true. My Dad used to say to me, "If you tell a lie enough, then you will actually start to believe it." If you believe your own exaggerated story, it becomes too challenging to make good judgments on how to learn from your dilemma, fix what is happening, and move on to accomplish your desired goal.

Whether we're dealing with a symptom of stress or exaggerating our situation, we need to understand the next and immediate action to take. If we are exaggerating, we need to stop.

Now. If we are contending with a stressor that overwhelms us, we need to take courage and remember that there is always light at the end of the tunnel. While this is not a physical step, it is certainly a positive mental action. I offer some steps at the end of this chapter along these lines.

Comfort Zones

Fear is like an invisible pair of arms squeezing you, holding you back. Imagine trying to run a race like that. You try to run, but no matter how hard you push, you barely go anywhere. This is how fear operates. In one area, we might be progressing, but in another, fears could be blocking our progress.

Many people adapt. They live in a way that doesn't make them face their fears. These people may even feel fearless – what fears? They have sealed off the situations that bring fear to them. They won't go there, no matter what. That is how they live, year after year… a classic comfort zone.

When you are inside the comfort zone, you feel … well, comfortable. However, you can only progress within that comfort zone. Chances are, if you continue along this route, you will look back at life during your twilight years and lament the opportunities you missed, wishing you'd drawn the courage to experience some of them. Or, you will wake up one day with an urge you haven't felt in quite awhile, to do something you have not done before, something greater than what you've accomplished. In either case, now is a great time to take the first step – right out of your comfort zone. It may not feel comfortable; you may feel uncertain. You have to face your fears.

An example of a comfort zone might be someone who loves to listen to public speakers and glean insight and knowledge from them… as long as he or she doesn't have to speak. If the opportunity or need to speak in public arises for any reason, a fear response overcomes the person. He or she feels terrible emotionally and physically. Sweaty hands, stuttering, coughing fits, and perspiration in potentially embarrassing areas (under the arms, for example) are common physical responses.

One day, the person decides, *enough is enough 'I'm going to overcome my fear'*. Perhaps they join a Toastmasters club, or another speaking group. Maybe they take public speaking lessons. Or, they get up and put one word in front of the other. Just like cliff-jumping, it gets easier with each event – and the person realizes that there is a safety net below (water for cliff jumpers, appreciative audiences for speakers), rather than an endless fall into oblivion. By overcoming the fear, they can speak in front of audiences. Their comfort zone has just expanded.

People possess comfort zone type fears in many areas of life. Examples include:

- One partner quitting work to raise the kids – and the other fearing the impact of the ensuing lost income and added responsibility of being sole provider
- Changing careers or seeking a promotion
- Starting a new relationship, or being willing to 'ask someone out'
- Buying a home
- Moving to a new city or state, away from family and long-time friends
- Asking for a pay rise
- Pursuing a big deal or a major goal
- Mustering the courage to say "Good morning" to someone you don't know
- Having children (and related fears of affordability, added workload, lack of sleep, change in lifestyle, etc.)
- Going overseas to visit historic and cultural sites; related issues of airport security, making flights on time, being victimized by crime, etc.

One final note: when you find any number of reasons to rationalize or justify not moving forward, that means you are touching the edge of your comfort zone. Break through it; make it happen for yourself.

Perception Is Everything

In order to master fear and stress, we need to address our perceptions about life situations. Perception is a reality to us. When we perceive something to be real, it is real to us, even if the rest of the world does not see it the same way. When we have an unbalanced perspective, our perceptions create more stress. It is vitally important to get our perceptions balanced if we want to master our stress level, our stressors, and our fears.

You may have heard of the acronym for fear–False Evidence Appearing Real–and similar descriptions. However, fear is really the *perception* that you will experience something more negative than positive, something which will hurt more than please.

Positives and negatives take on a slightly different meaning in this discussion. A magnet includes a positive and negative end. You can't have two positive ends or two negative ends. With a book, you have a beginning and an end, a front and a back, an up and a down, left and right, a start and a stop. Good novelists know that they can't keep their readers "up" the entire time, no matter how positive the book. Likewise, even in the darkest horror and fantasy books, you find moments of levity and humor to lift people up. No matter what you face, there are always two sides, a pro and con.

How do we see both sides? By opening our minds. In Chapter 2, I presented tools to show the different sides and how we can work these to our advantage to balance our perception, assisting us in achieving greater serenity, relaxation and happiness.

I have a brother, a few years older than me. He always invited me to do things with him, even to the point that he let me hang out with his friends. However, this same brother used to beat me up quite regularly. I considered him a real jerk because of the pain that I suffered at his hands. I didn't think he was a good brother at all. In fact, I came to fear him.

Ten years later, his lovely wife was talking to me about why he used to hit me. He told her that he had received word that I was being beaten up at school and couldn't defend myself. He had tried to talk to me about fighting back against these guys who had been attacking me. He thought I was afraid to retaliate. In his mind, talking to me didn't work, so he thought beating me up might help. It seemed like a good idea to him at the time, since he thought it would toughen me and teach me some fighting skills. It wasn't that I couldn't stand up for myself, but I just wasn't a violent person and I never liked fighting. I could if I needed to, but it just wasn't my thing. I preferred to play sports and socialize.

The point to this example? My fear-based perception was wrong. I thought my brother was bullying me, when in fact he was also acting from *kindness and concern*. He thought that he was helping me to toughen up and stand up for myself.

In another example, a client, Bruce, thought he had landed a job. His interview was dynamic, and he was confident things would pan out his way. But when he got knocked back, fear set in, along with its never-ending questions: "How long will I be unemployed?" "How will we pay our rent?" "Why wasn't I good enough this time? Will I be good enough next time?" "What will my wife think of me now?"

At first, things did go badly. He had to borrow money from a friend to pay the rent. However, an opportunity opened up that was actually better than the previous one. This time, he got the job, and it turned into a long-term, highly successful (and very well paid) career. His source of pain (not landing the job) actually brought something greater into his life - an even better career.

Fearing the Unknown

One of our greatest collective fears is the unknown. We like to feel in control of what will happen next, but because we only have limited control on future events and circumstances–if at all– we fear the future will not pan out the way we would like it to. We hope and wish for things to turn out well, but often consider only the worst-case scenario. Hollywood has made countless billions in the past 20 years with movies tapping into this fear: *Armageddon, Day After Tomorrow, 2012,* the *X-Men* movies, etc.

Too often, we look for and expect guarantees in life: we won't get hurt in this relationship; the business venture will be a million-dollar success; we will live a stress-free life without health issues (because we can't imagine living *with* a health issue). When we are not open to different possible outcomes, we set ourselves up to suffer more stress than needed. There are things that we can do to minimize our risks, such as researching a market, getting to really know a person before entering a committed relationship, exercising often, eating right and taking supplements, but these actions only increase the chances it will go our way. Nothing in life is really guaranteed, aside from death.

Many of my clients are scared of opening up to a committed relationship, due to their past experiences. Many have experienced deep hurt, endured a cheating or dishonest partner, or feel they can't trust their loved one anymore. They fear the same problems will happen again, and hurt even more, so they protect themselves by building walls around their hearts. My job is to help them to understand that their past difficulties do not need to paint their future. Many have gone on to have fulfilling relationships.

When you want something, chase it with the hope everything will work out. At the same time, prepare for what you will need if things don't turn out the way you planned. Insurance is a great example of expecting the best and preparing for the worst. My Dad used to be a life insurance salesman. He said something I found rather amusing: "When you buy life insurance, you are betting that you will die, the insurance company is betting that you won't, and you are doing everything to help them win." This goes with every type of insurance. These are probably the only bets you are more than happy to lose. You are expecting the best, but in case the worst does happen, you are prepared.

Some future possibilities are likely to occur, such as a child going to college, or paying for your daughter's wedding. You don't wait until your child finishes high school to say, "Oh, I'd better start saving for college". Instead, you put a little aside each week or month so that you are prepared for the sticker shock when the time comes.

The same holds true for retirement. Start saving now and putting a little aside so that you will be financially secure in the future.

To slightly modify the old saying, "Work for the best but prepare for the worst." This is not to cast a negative, self-sabotaging spell on your efforts. It's merely a reminder that we don't know for sure what's to come. Likewise, no use fearing something that hasn't happened yet. That's a waste of emotional energy. Just plan for various possibilities.

Facing Fears

Courage is the ability to do something that initially frightens us–sometimes, greatly. It is not the absence of fear, but the ability to face that fear and move forward. The cliff jumper practiced courage by taking the 10-meter leap. It might have been fool's courage, but it was courage nonetheless. By the time Austrian extreme sportsman Felix Baumgartner jumped out of a plane from the 'edge of space' in October 2012, 39 kilometers above New Mexico, he had taken hundreds of preparatory jumps, some as high as 25 kilometers. Still, he felt fear. What if his pressurized suit sprung a leak at 30 kilometers altitude, while he was plummeting down faster than the speed of sound?

If we break it down a little further, we realize we face a lot more than simple fear. We also face the discouragement, sadness, helplessness and hopelessness that we might have experienced previously when we caved. This time, we produce a different result. We do whatever needs to be done. We face all the different mental or emotional "gremlins" and affirm, "I can do it anyway." By adopting this way of thinking, we move forward and accomplish the goal. (At this point, it is good to congratulate yourself and do something nurturing and self-caring, to soothe your mind and heart after your efforts.)

I had a client that was downright frightened to ask for what she wanted. She was afraid to ask people to help her, or to see if she could help them. She would never ask for money, or anything else. She hated the idea of asking for anything. It petrified her. There were times, of course, when she truly needed help, or felt the need to help others, or needed to earn money. Almost everything required her to ask someone for something – unless she wanted to sit and wait for things to land in her lap. And that wasn't working so well. What could she do without the courage to move forward?

One day in the clinic, she told me that she needed to call someone to ask for something, but was too scared. I found out who it was, dialed the number, and handed her the phone. She didn't have any time to feel the fear, because when she put the phone to her ear, the person on the other end had picked up. The two spoke, and with some persistence on my part, she eventually asked for what she wanted. The other person was happy to oblige. After we hung up, my client burst into tears. Throughout her phone conversation, she waited and expected to hear the same rejection to which she had become accustomed while growing up.

Most of her life, she had not been given the things for which she had asked. Her family filled her with the belief that if she received something, another person was missing out. She was ridiculed for asking. She blamed herself for the pain her parents felt (or so she perceived) when she asked for things they couldn't afford. It got to the point where she stopped asking. In this instance, in my office, she faced her fear. Now, she released an overwhelming amount of emotion stored up from this part of her life.

In a somewhat similar situation, a client grew up in a poor home, as far as money was concerned. One of the things she remembered her mother saying often was, "Those who ask, do not receive" or "Those who ask, do not get." My client went into adulthood believing that if she asked, she would not receive, so I had to teach her that she would not receive only if she *didn't* ask. It took lot of work to help her overcome this deeply ingrained belief. I encouraged her to call people when she needed to ask for something. After doing this numerous times, she noticed that it was starting to get easier and easier. She still felt the fear that she was going to get rejected, that "No" would be the answer. She felt fear, discouragement, anguish and insecurity about each call, but she still took the phone and dialed. She found that it wasn't as hurtful as she thought. She made her life easier – and broke a fear that had crippled her.

We need to recognize opportunity. Fear is really just an opportunity to grow. If we see it like that, then we can look at all these different stresses and fears as a way to be courageous and grow in different areas of life.

Overcoming Fear–And Moving Forward

Look back at your life, the stress you have been through, and how you have dealt with different circumstances and people. Look at the achievements of which you are most proud, like earning a degree, developing a trade, or excelling in a sport.

Notice something in common? In all cases, you worked through stress and overcame initial fears, some of them minor, some of them intense. Learn to realize how much you grew from each stress and challenge, to see the benefits of stress. When you evaluate your life like this, you will find that every experience has actually been helpful. You will also start to see that you likely overcame a fear in each area–failing an exam, being cut by your team, hurting your hand on a machine, and on and on–and still you moved forward.

When pursuing your goals, there are two ways to arrive at your destination:

1) Take it slowly, assuring yourself of little to no stress. The problem? It takes forever to get there – if you do at all–and reflects a fear of stepping out of your comfort zone.

2) Intensify the journey. Step outside your comfort zone, deal with the stress and displeasure as it occurs, accomplish the goal you have set, and feel good about what you have achieved.

Let's look at these approaches as they pertain to weightlifting. You can lift small weights to strengthen and tone your muscles, but if your goal is bodybuilding then you must intensify the effort. Instead of lifting 45 kg. (100 lbs.), you must lift 90 kg. (200 lbs.) or more. You will perform fewer reps, but your workouts will be more intense. You will achieve the desired result. The same principle holds true for life. The more stress we can handle in a growth situation, the faster we adapt to handle more of what life can and does throw our way.

Why do we put ourselves through so much stress? Why do we endure it? Why do we keep finding ourselves in stressful situations? The positive answer is to gain knowledge from our experience and utilize it. Knowledge is far more than what we learn in school. The most important knowledge we acquire comes through direct experience.

I saw an interview with Donald Trump in which he spoke about how doing business had always been so easy for him. Then, after his bull rush through the 1980s, when his American real estate properties were valued greater than any U.S. citizen, he lost everything. That put him under a lot of stress. During this time, he said, he grew the most, on both personal and business levels. I'm sure he looks back at it now and sees the ensuing bankruptcy issues as a very important part of his life, which further sharpened him to again become a global business titan.

Stress and fear are growth experiences. When we feel these in association with our comfort zone, we can embrace the situation and carry on, knowing it is part of our journey. The things you fear may not be so bad in the long run, as Trump learned from his bankruptcy. These situations don't happen often, but when they do, learn from them and prepare to reap their related benefits. Think about things from a logical perspective and don't allow fear to run – or ruin – your life.

Techniques for Conquering Fear

Whether finding better employment, being assertive, making new friends, getting to know someone you'd like to date, making a big financial decision, starting a business venture, public speaking, or moving to a new area, if you take steps outside your comfort zone of skill, security, knowledge and ability–something bigger than normal–then you will feel fear. Along with that will come its unwelcome sidekick … stress.

When you learn from your experiences and overcome your stresses, you empower yourself. You are no longer stressed from those situations, as you know how to deal with them appropriately. You have eliminated another potential source of stress. In this way, you attract greater peace of mind. You live with greater happiness and joy, and less frustration. When these dynamics occur, you have successfully "let go" of a fear or stressor.

When you feel fear, remember that moving past your comfort zone is a part of progress. While it might seem harder initially, in the long run, the benefits of overcoming fear far outweigh the effort involved. As the saying goes, "Feel the fear and do it anyway." It takes just as much work to keep on hiding from something, as it does to face it and deal with it. So you may as well deal with it and reap all the benefits!

If you want to achieve a certain goal, but it lies beyond your comfort zone, break it down into steps. Instead of being overwhelmed with the task, take steps like these:

1. Remember that for every problem, there is a solution

2. Realize you are only presented with challenges that you are capable of overcoming

3. Acknowledge that when your mind is in worst-case scenario mode, what you think and feel is blown out of proportion 99% of the time, and is not likely to happen

Now ask yourself, "What can I do to overcome this?" Break it down into actionable steps. Make each step a little more of a reach on your part, a little more difficult to attain.

In private consultations, I quickly help clients uncover the driving force behind their fear (often an earlier trauma) and dissolve the emotion around it, to weaken the impact of the fear on their present lives. This often transforms the emotional charge. Once that happens, they can take action steps much easier. One way of acknowledging the deeper reason behind your fear is to use the questioning techniques in Chapter 1. When you are aware of a fear, ask yourself "Why does that bother me?" to uncover the deeper reason. Then ask "Why does *that* (the deeper reason) bother me?" Usually after 3 or 4 rounds of asking this question, the real motivation behind the surface fear is evident. You can then mentally separate the current situation from that fear response.

When I set out to write this book, the whole idea scared me. I felt some serious, tangible fear. How was I going to take my expertise and experiences, and write 80,000 words about it? Believe me, my mind was cranking up a good worst-case scenario–that I would never get to the final chapter!

I set off by addressing my fear, using the steps above. I dissolved the emotional constraints around my goal by deciding I would move logically to organize the materials, then bring in stories to illustrate them, and then start writing. That resolved my first fear: getting everything together. Then, I broke that giant 80,000-word perceived mountain into chapters. As you may have noticed, I took it even further, and created sections within the chapters. I kept my eyes on the road, one chapter at a time.

What was my most important and courageous step? Typing the first sentence. Taking the first step. If you don't type that first sentence, or walk into that office to ask for a pay rise, how will you ever know what might happen? Reaffirm to yourself that you are worth it, that you can do it, and carry on. That is the way to a fulfilling life, in which stress is a valuable ally, not an enemy.

Chapter 10: Peace from Within

It sounds like the simplest state of being. We wake up and pass through our day in a state of peace and joy, viewing the good in everyone and everything. We feel strong, self-assured and serene, confident that every decision we make will be good, right, or at least take us in a positive direction. When difficulties come our way, we ground ourselves into this deep place, quiet our minds, and reach a solution. Such a harmonious state brings with it lasting happiness. And stress? *What* stress?

Inner peace is our birthright; we possessed it when we were born. That being the case, why do we spend many years seeking it, thousands of dollars visiting yoga/meditation retreats or therapists trying to tap into it, hundreds more dollars on books to learn systems to reclaim it, and untold sums dealing with the medical effects of not having it? What happens to tip the scales on inner peace? When and why do we allow doubt, fear, limitation, worry and stress into our lives? Why is it so easy to say, "Peace be with you," yet so hard to apply it? How do we get back to our birthright? *Will* we get back to it?

Unfortunately, this inner battle plays out on a global scale. So many people are petitioning for peace, crying, begging and praying for it. And yet, since 2001 (and for a long time before then), large parts of our world have been at war. So many people are looking for world peace, looking for someone to bring it to them. Yet, conflict never seems to end. World peace is inner peace on a global scale. It concerns every one of us possessing and expressing peace from within, and reflecting our peace to the rest of the world, one person at a time. Until everyone is willing to put the effort into loving themselves and sustaining inner peace, there will never be lasting world peace.

We have to be willing to go within and actively find peace. When we do, and it permeates our lives, we reach the ultimate purpose of this book: a stress-proof life, in which every situation is addressed promptly and on its own terms by self-love, self-knowing, conflict resolution, relationship building and with a deep personal sense of peace and fairness.

Let's look at some of the forces that work against inner peace, and then discuss how we can attain that state that seamlessly merges wisdom, childlike innocence and deep compassion, empathy, and contentment.

Enemies of Inner Peace

What prevents inner peace? We've spent much of this book addressing stressors and the state of being stressed out. Those make inner peace harder to come by. Two huge culprits are guilt and shame, polar opposites to the deep self-love that anchors inner peace. When you feel deep guilt and shame, not only do turmoil and doubt dominate your thoughts and feelings, but you're living in a self-absorbed place. Inner peace isn't self-absorption at all. It is the act of living from a centered, balanced space in which you are eminently comfortable with yourself and able to touch others in a positive way.

Other enemies of peace include fear, pride, anger, hate, resentment, revenge, and insecurity. All of these can take over and bring a feeling of turmoil. That leads to insecurity, conflict and feelings of lack or low self-worth. These seven negative emotions often work together to send us on an out-of-control spiral, to the depths of despair and hopelessness.

When taken to the extreme, fear and pride can lead to inner and outer war. Let's go back to an example we are well aware of, Adolf Hitler. He exercised the incredible power of his own personal pride to proclaim his Aryan people a superior race. Why? He greatly feared the Jews taking over Europe financially. His fear was just as real and profound as his pride. The two merged into a mighty personal and national obsession with exterminating Jews, and eventually anyone that disagreed with him. Most of the world was dragged into World War II because of Hitler's misplaced pride that he and his people were superior to all others. *One man's misplaced pride.*

On an everyday level, fear and misplaced pride can lead to disharmony from within and with those around us. We fear that someone else will receive or acquire something that we will not. If they get it, we won't. Or, our prideful thinking will kick in, causing us to see ourselves as superior. We may tear others down verbally. We often show our fear and pride when we attack other people and what they have accomplished, or when we accuse them of not achieving a feat alone because they had to get help.

Ironically, this line of attack comes from insecurity. Our prideful actions compensate for our inner lack of self-respect. Because of our fear and pride, we often take actions and make decisions that are quite different from what we first intended. We get upset with ourselves and feel guilty because we realize how hurtful and unkind we have been. We may push this guilt aside mentally, but it really gets stuffed inside and adds to our lack of self-respect.

Everyone possesses these enemies of peace within themselves. How we act and respond, or react, when potentially negative situations occur, points to our state of mind, and our inner peace. When we react, we do not consider the consequences of our actions. However, when we *act* or *respond,* we think about what to do and make more rational decisions about the right steps to take. Think *pro*actively, not *re*actively.

Sometimes, when we allow these emotions to control us instead of us controlling them, we become embroiled in feuds. These feuds can happen between two siblings, a parent and child, or both parents–with siblings taking sides. This can disintegrate into a war within a family. What is war, after all, but a dispute or disagreement over philosophies, policies or desired possessions between people who happen to be in a position to order their armies to fight a battle? War is disagreement blown way out of proportion. A family feud is a war within a family.

We need to learn to deal with our emotions and be in control of them at all times. The enemies of peace are the emotions over which we don't take control.

More on Pride

We are taught from a young age to be loyal to our country. We are taught to love its heritage, values, culture, citizens, and the opportunities it affords us. This is a good thing. However, some people take this love of country too far, into prideful thinking, in which they believe themselves better than others because of where they are from. They will claim that it's patriotism, but there's nothing patriotic about it. This is runaway pride.

Patriotism is an attitude of loyalty and willingness to defend one's country and values when needed. Pride comes from the insecurity that maybe your country is not so good, or it's so superior that you attack others, whether verbally or physically. Patriotism defends, and pride attacks. This seems to be a problem in many countries.

So many of us are taught from a young age that we are better than our neighbors, the kids at school, or those with different colored skin or accents. As soon as someone introduces an idea or policy that isn't in line with our prejudiced (pre-judged) thoughts, then we attack and try to tear them down.

Two Types of Peace

To better understand the concept of living from a state of inner peace by having peace from within, let's examine the two types of peace. The first is **peace of mind**. Most of us seek greater peace of mind on a daily basis. Our desire increases as more external forces, the things happening around us, affect our lives. These might include the economy, jobs, personal finances, war, family issues, and a variety of situations. They can cause turmoil within our mind, creating a lack of peace. Consequently, we lose our inner peace.

We sometimes think this is a permanent loss, but as the saying goes, "This too shall pass…" It is only temporary. It only remains as long as the external stress is there. For example, if a tiger walks into the room, you will have a stress response. Your gut will tighten as you question if you will survive. As soon as the tiger leaves the room, provided you are not in its stomach, you can run over, lock the door and shake for a few minutes. Then you do not need to stress about it anymore; the initial threat is gone. In a more ordinary example than an encounter in the Bengal jungle, suppose our finances aren't great and we need to pay some bills. Where will the money come from? A sure way to overcome this stress in the future is to learn how to manage your finances. The first rule to restore financial peace of mind? Spend less than you earn. It may not be easy. It may even be impossible–or so you think. You may have to give up unnecessary wants and desires, but you can do it. Then start a savings program, as we discussed in Chapter 7. There are things you can do to resolve this stress and restore peace of mind.

The second type of peace is **peace of consciousness**. Inner turmoil will impact peace of consciousness. Those who possess peace of consciousness love themselves regardless of mistakes they make – or have made. The extent of our peace of consciousness draws from the things that we do, think and say that cause either a settled or unsettled mind. The first way to maintain peace of consciousness is by doing the right things. If we do something wrong, we need to correct our mistake by going back and sorting it out with whomever was involved.

When we do not possess peace of consciousness, our problems can feel relentless. They're open for business 24/7. Guilty feelings about a past event will pop up every now and then. An old source of shame might come back. What about the money you still owe a friend from a year ago? Things eat at us because our larger consciousness wants what the soul wants– peace. That restless, unsettled, undeviating state will remain until it is corrected.

What if we don't want to deal with these nagging concerns? Some choose to mask or hide them. Drinking too much alcohol, taking drugs, excessive T.V. watching, oversleeping and playing PlayStation until the wee hours, night after night, are among the faces on these masks. These can help for a little while, but when the show ends, you wake up or become sober, the core problems are still waiting – just where you left them.

Why do our problems circle back to mess with our inner peace? *To remind us that we have not dealt with them.* We can't change the past, but we can correct some of the outcomes. We can sort them out as best we can and make amends where possible. This allows us to be at peace with ourselves and to move on. Even if you hurt someone and they don't want to let it go, as long as you have done everything possible to make amends, then you can move on in peace. Making amends is an expression of self-forgiveness. Whether or not the other person forgives you is their business.

A restless consciousness can be a gift. It may not feel that way, but few feelings match the peace that results from successfully dealing with the source of the unease. You feel more peaceful emotionally, mentally, and spiritually. You come to a happy, balanced, neutral state, one of constant calmness and poise, no matter the situation.

Even when you have peace of consciousness, you can (and will) continue to experience disruptions. But now, you respond in a clearer state. If you practice this, and then touch one other person at a time with your deep serenity, then you will help to bring about world peace.

When I was a small child, my family was very well to do. As I was starting school, we experienced great financial challenges. I watched the other kids eat their really nice food and snacks, while I turned up with just a sandwich. I felt hard done by, wondering why I didn't get nice snacks, too.

I decided to start sneaking into the classroom when it was empty, and helping myself to the nice foods in other students' bags. Eventually, I got caught. When my mother found out, I told her that it was not true; it was just another way for the teacher to pick on me. Because I had been picked on by some of the teachers, it was easy to convince my Mom that this was another instance of their harassment.

For years, I held the guilt and shame of not telling the truth. My parents had taught me to be honest. I beat myself up over it, and struggled to keep those occasional guilty thoughts out of my mind. This shame and guilt didn't come from stealing food. I had spoken to the kid from whom I had taken it and fixed it up with him. It arose from being dishonest. Fifteen years later, when I was 22, I finally came clean and told my Mom the truth. It had lingered and weighed on my conscience for almost three quarters of my life at that point. She was a little disappointed in me, but the guilt and shame were finally gone. A weight had been lifted off my shoulders. I finally had peace of consciousness.

If you still have something unresolved in your life, now is the time to fix it up and free yourself from the burden. Allow yourself the peace of consciousness that you really desire – and deserve.

Facing Problems

How many times have problems, situations or dilemmas fallen into our lives–and we swept them under the rug? Think of how often you have pulled up that imaginary carpet and whisked a problem or two under there. We think we're making our day easier, keeping peace with our spouses or kids, or dusting away an issue that will never return. This is instant gratification and instant comfort thinking. It's also the wrong way to think. Life doesn't work that way. If it's not resolved, it *will* come back, which makes procrastination one of the greatest threats to lasting inner peace. Procrastination extends its toxic force in two ways. First, we know how to fix a problem, but we put off doing it because of a real or imagined fear. The fears of rejection, being resented, and getting into trouble of some sort lead the way. One or more of these fears holds us back. Sometimes, we procrastinate for a few minutes or hours. (At other times, we hold onto it for 15 years, as I did. I feared my Mom's disappointment and possible punishment.) Consequently, we stifle the peace we would like. We do not move on. We idle.

The same predicament often happens when we want to start something new. We fear failure or being wrong. We really want to move forward, but procrastinate because of these fears. At the end of the day, we never find out if we would have succeeded or failed. This weakens our confidence in doing the things we want to do. We suffer more than had we attempted and failed. Again, we do not attain that peace we want so badly.

The second face of procrastination involves starting and finishing things. Our minds race about what needs to be done. The big question is, will we ever leave the starting blocks? If you want to start something and don't, the "what if?" question dogs your consciousness like a pack of starving dingos. It never lets up. Most people are great project starters. The number of great finishers is far fewer.

Your mind likes complete pictures. If you start something and do not finish it, you may think about why it's not done and the actions, time and energy you need to complete the project. If you have many unfinished projects, then your mind spreads itself thin to accommodate them, making it nearly impossible to concentrate efficiently. It is like sitting in a coffee shop or café, trying to penetrate the background noise to focus on one specific thing. All of those projects demand your time and attention. When you feel stymied, procrastination sets in, and peace becomes as evasive as a midnight burglar.

One day, I was helping my brother deal with issues he was having with his children. I suggested some steps he could take to help his children along in the process. He didn't like my delivery. When I left, I knew he was not completely happy with me. It wasn't what I said, but the way I said it. I respect my brother greatly. He is fun to be around, very caring, kind and nonjudgmental, but I avoided seeing him because of my fear he would still be upset with me. Our children loved being around each other. That too stopped, because I hadn't taken them around. My children were living with the effect of my choice.

I needed to speak with my brother and clear the air, but I was still concerned with his reaction. When we spoke, he said he was annoyed at me for about half an hour. That was it. Afterwards, he put my suggestions into practice, and they helped. For three months, I sat in discomfort and a lack of peace. He sat in that state for thirty minutes. If I had not procrastinated about clearing the air with him, my kids would have played with his kids during those three lost months. After finally facing my fear and talking to him, I gained the peace that I sought.

When you realize you need to fix something in your life, don't put it off unnecessarily. Definitely don't rush in (while still stressed) and make the problem worse. But once you know you can at least partially resolve the problem, get to work. It deepens your inner peace.

World Peace in Michael Jackson's song "Man in the Mirror", he sings, "I'm starting with the man in the mirror. I'm asking him to change his ways. No message could have been any clearer. If you want to make the world a better place, take a look at yourself and then make a change."

If we want to find peace in the world, our search must start from within ourselves. As I mentioned, world peace is inner peace on a grand scale. We need to evaluate ourselves, and be honest about our evaluations. When we want to make changes, we need to do more than focusing on our strengths and brushing aside our weaknesses.

Many gurus today will tell you not to worry about what you have done wrong, just focus on your strengths. Or they will say you should focus on attaining peace and bliss; that alone will solve your many problems. The trouble with this teaching is, we are not loaves of bread. We can't love ourselves in slices. We are whole beings, with positives and negatives, strengths and weaknesses. We need to acknowledge and accept both in order to rediscover peace within. We need to acknowledge both sides evenly. Acknowledge our strengths and build on them, then acknowledge our weaknesses and work on them until they, too, become strengths.

Michael Jordan said, "My attitude is that if you push me towards something that you think is a weakness, then I will turn that perceived weakness into a strength." He would work on a weakness until it became a strength; that way, opponents could not use a weakness against him. When Jordan came into the NBA, he wasn't a strong defender. When he left the NBA, he was regarded as one of greatest defensive players of all time. Notice that I didn't mention offense, for which Jordan is best known. Jordan was willing to acknowledge where he could improve–defensively. Because of that, he became what many believe to be the greatest basketball player of all time.

If you don't acknowledge your faults or shortcomings, someone else will. They may try to capitalize on them, whether in business, sport or relationships. It is important for you to acknowledge and work on them yourself and put yourself in a better place in all areas of life.

A lot of people want peace, but need the courage to find it. We need to go within, face ourselves, take on and dismantle our demons, and attain and build the resulting peace. We often seem to be our own harshest judges. We also need to be our own biggest fans.

Sharing Peace

Now that we understand the two types of peace, we are in a position to help others. Understand that everyone's journey is individual, and that it is important for them to learn lessons so that they can grow. Still, we can contribute greatly to that. You never know if you are going to be the one that will say the right words, offer the friendly smile that touches someone the right way, or become the influence someone needs to make a decision to move forward. The key is to put yourself in that position. When you do, your sense of inner peace will soar, as will your self-empowerment and your ability to help empower others.

Speaking of soaring, the majestic eagle is one of my favorite animals. I love learning about them and how they navigate the skies. I'm always amazed at how they help their young learn to fly. They push their young either off a high tree or mountain, and give them lessons in flying. If the young eagle does not fly, and instead starts falling toward a certain death, the parent races down and catches the young eaglet in time to repeat the lesson. Eventually, the young bird flies for itself, but it needs that push from its parent.

We do not know for sure if our little push in the right direction will propel the other person past what they are going through, and bring them some of the peace they are seeking. Sometimes, we will feel discouraged, with voices telling us that we can't do it, or that we can't help this person, or save the world: "What a waste of your time! This person doesn't even want your help!" This happens. We just need to look within ourselves and our motivations, and remind ourselves of the value we offer those who do want help.

Once you respect what you have overcome, you may be drawn to others experiencing the same or similar trials. Or, they may be drawn to you. Use your experience to help others overcome their challenges and learn from their stresses even faster. Your experience then benefits others as well as yourself.

Tell them about the light at the end of the tunnel, and then help them recognize it for themselves.

Remember what I said in Chapter 7 about giving charitably? In addition to my suggestion of giving 10% to a charity of your choice, the benefits of giving a bit of your time to make others' lives easier is of equal or greater benefit. Not to mention a fun, joyful experience–and one from which you will learn as well. An easy way to do this is by sharing your experiences. Share your wins and losses, the things that did and didn't work, so others can learn from the mistakes you made, emulate the techniques you used or choices you made to get it right, and shortcut a painful part of the learning curve that you experienced. In this way, empower others. This dynamic happens every time you attend a seminar, workshop or other learning forum. The seminar or workshop leader is typically someone with many years of experience at his/her skill and profession. Most had mentors who showed them the ropes. While these people earn some money for their workshops, a much more noble drive has brought them to stand in front of you: the desire to share their experiences, good and bad, and to give you tools to improve your skills more quickly. They are empowering you, almost as if they plugged themselves into your skin and gave you an electrical charge of empowerment.

You can do this, too. I suggest you do. When sharing your experience, be honest. Don't exaggerate your story. It's inspiring as-is. If someone comes to you for help, they see learning points in your story and experience. Be yourself. Be authentic.

Not everyone will run up to you with open arms and say, "Give me advice. Help me move forward." Some people will like you and others won't; that's life. As for the ones that won't like you, I have a quick question: Who cares? For those who find you engaging, wouldn't you prefer to be yourself instead of feeling as if you have to be someone else? As British playwright and poet Oscar Wilde said, "Be yourself; everyone else is already taken."

This reminds me of a client with whom I worked, a big lady with low self-esteem. While growing up, her Dad told her she was fat, ugly and no one would ever want her. After she came to me, and I listened to her experience, we set some goals, and helped her overcome some self-sabotaging actions and stresses she typically brought into every goal she tried to achieve. When it came to her weight, we didn't set a number, but a size and image with which she felt comfortable. Part of the "homework" I assigned was to buy an outfit in the goal size, and put it somewhere where she would see it every day.

After a period of time, and after many setbacks, she achieved her goal. Her Dad still told her she was ugly, not worth anything and that no one would want her, but he couldn't say she was fat anymore. We continued to work on eliminating the stress she felt when he voiced his opinion. She got to a point where his opinion didn't matter anymore. I showed her that he was insecure about his own weight, health and self-worth, and how that insecurity made him attack her. Her confidence grew so much that she had the courage to tell him to keep his opinion to himself. Today, he does. Afterwards, she shared her experience with family, friends and colleagues. Many of them started to take action to improve their own health. Some even came to me for the same help I had given her.

Another example involves a friend of my wife. He suffered a major stroke and was not expected to survive the night. Six months later, he was back at work, living a pretty normal life. He started a website to help stroke survivors struggling through similar experiences. He has also authored a book, outlining the stresses and triumphs he faced on his road to recovery. He inspires stroke survivors all over the world.

My final example concerns the late Steve Jobs. Nine years after he and Steve Wozniak built Apple Computers from scratch, he was forced to resign when the Board of Directors would not subscribe to his vision about the company's future possibilities. On Google, there are links to speeches Jobs made in the early

1980s, discussing a world of iPads, iPods, iCloud and iTunes, as if it were already happening. He just didn't have the available technology. But he had the vision–one that Apple's board couldn't imagine, let alone see.

Jobs left and created NeXT Computer. (Tim Berners-Lee invented the World Wide Web on a NeXT computer.) In 1986, Jobs paid *Star Wars* creator George Lucas $5 million to purchase the graphics division of Lucasfilm Ltd. He later renamed it Pixar. How good was this investment? When Jobs sold Pixar to Disney in 2006, he received $7.4 *billion,* according to the *Wall Street Journal.*

By 1997, Apple had suffered enough creatively, and only held a 3% share of the personal computer marketplace. They brought back Jobs after a 12-year absence. He took Apple from a struggling, $10-per-share company to one of the most innovative and important companies in the world, with products helping define *seven* industries and share prices peaking at $702 in September 2012. As of March 2013, according to *Fortune Magazine*, Apple had $145 billion in cash–or nearly twice the on-hand currency in the United States Treasury. And, yes, Jobs' vision of an "i" world came to bear in fullest glory.

While Jobs was known for being taciturn and sometimes even cruel, as well as doggedly competitive and protective of Apple products, he always helped others through his example. His speech to the Stanford University 2005 graduating class is considered one of the greatest commencement addresses ever made. It's subject? Don't give up, don't give in to difficulties, embrace your challenges, face your fears, deal with your stresses… and pass on what you've learned to others.

Throughout history, the most successful pioneers, voyagers and travelers have never been the fastest. The best blazed a trail making it easier for others to pass through. We can use the depth of our experience, our wisdom to overcome stress, and our example to create a model of how to live to make life easier for those who follow us. This will help them find peace and tranquility even faster – the ultimate gift we can offer toward a life beyond stress.

Final Word

Of all the skills we gain in life, learning to handle and resolve stress is one of the most essential. With the tools in this book you are now more capable of both resolving your specific stressors and feeling more happiness and joy in life. Use the tools one chapter, one day at a time, to gradually change your life. Invest the comparatively small amount of time needed to implement the strategies you have learned. After all, the life with less stress that you have been looking for is yours for the taking. You deserve it! Make it yours!

References and bibliography

1. William Glasser, MD. (1997). *Choice Theory. Interviewing Skills for Helping Professionals.* Association for Applied Control Theory Australia. 2012

2. *Marriage and Crude Marriage Rates.* United Nations Statistical Division (UNSTAT). 2011
   Divorce and Crude Divorce Rates. United Nations Statistical Division (UNSTAT). 2011

3. Barron, Robert A; Richardson, Deborah R. (1994). Human Aggression. *Perspectives in Social Psychology.* 2nd edition.

4. *Psychology Today.* The Grateful Brain: The Neuroscience of Giving Thanks. Alex Korb, PhD. Nov 20, 2012.; King, MW. (2002). *Tyrosine-Derived Neurotransmitters.* Indiana State University.; *Dopamine.* Monica Siegenthaler, Davidson College. 2003 http://www.bio.davidson.edu/Courses/Molbio/MolStudents/spring2003/Siegenthaler/home.html

5. Oxford Dictionary. 2014. http://www.oxforddictionaries.com/definition/english/sacrifice

6. Collins Dictionary. 2014. http://www.collinsdictionary.com/dictionary/english/sacrifice

7. *Wasted: How America Is Losing up to 40 Percent of its Food from Farm to Fork to Landfill.* Dana Gunders. Natural Resources Defence Council. 2012. http://www.nrdc.org/food/files/wasted-food-ip.pdf

8. *Global Food Losses and Food Waste: Extent, Causes and Prevention.* Food and Agriculture Organization of the United Nations. 2011. http://www.fao.org/docrep/014/mb060e/mb060e00.pdf

9. *The Holy Bible*, Authorized King James Version.

10. *The Holy Bible*, Authorized King James Version.

11. *Water Supply, Sanitation and Hygiene Development.* World Health Organization. 2014.
http://www.who.int/water_sanitation_health/hygiene/en/

12. *Global Health Observatory: Slum Residence.* World Health Organization. 2014.
http://www.who.int/gho/urban_health/determinants/slum_residen ce_text/en/; *Press Briefing by Special Rapporteur on Right to Adequate Housing.* United Nations. 2005.
http://www.un.org/News/briefings/docs/2005/kotharibrf050511.d oc.htm

In Praise of DeStress To Success
by Leo Willcocks:

"In our work with star performers in many diverse organizations, we learned that the 'stars' experience stress differently than everyone else. Because of their deep commitment to a greater purpose and complete mastery of their job and environment, they experience less stress overall and handle it better when stresses are put on them. *DeStress to Success* gives everyone the tools to handle stress the way top performers handle stress, allowing everyone to become a star."

–Dr. William Seidman
CEO of Cerebyte, Inc. Author of *The Star Factor*

"Easy to read and hits the nail right on the head. This book is a must for anyone serious about creating higher self-esteem and eliminating stress."

-Jim Huling
Co-author of the #1 Wall Street Journal National Bestseller
The 4 Disciplines of Execution, Global Managing Consultant for Franklin Covey

"Dealing with stress and its effects is one of the biggest challenges we all face. If you want lasting peace and the ability to resolve stress for good, then *DeStress to Success* is the book for you."

-Dale Beaumont
Best-selling author of the *Secrets Exposed* Series

"If you find yourself stuck on the treadmill of life, feeling stressed day in day out, Leo Willcocks provides the answer you are looking for in his book *DeStress to Success*."

-Rick Frishman
PR maven, best-selling author and speaker, Publisher at Morgan James Publishing

"*DeStress to Success* shows Leo's deep understanding of human nature and how to turn self-sabotage into self-empowerment. If you have ever experienced stress or fear in your life this book is for you."

-Benjamin J. Harvey
Founder of Authentic Education